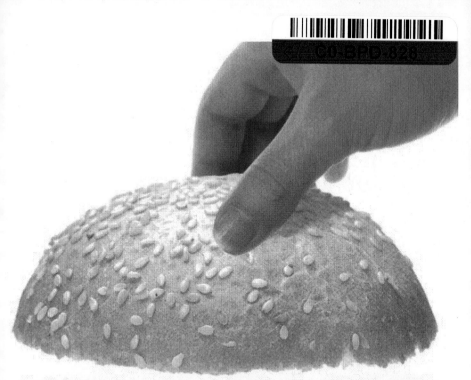

THE STORY YOU HAVEN'T BEEN TOLD
FAST FOOD VINDICATION
Lisa Tillinger Johansen, MS, RD

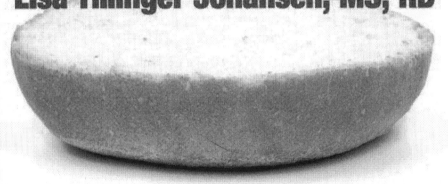

Yo Judy,
Here's to healthy eating!
Alisa Tillinger Johansen

To the three most important people in my life…
My beloved husband and best friend Roy, I couldn't have done it without you.

and

My wonderful parents, Jerry and Sherry, you are both sorely missed.

Acknowledgments

Many thanks are due to the executives and company representatives from the fast food and sit-down restaurants who were so generous with their time and observations. Jim Carras from the McDonald's Corporation was especially helpful. Eric Deardorff from PETA added much to my understanding of his organization's perspective.

Sarah Ross and Michael Tunison were my editors extraordinaire, and their guidance helped me immeasurably. Their intelligence, patience and good humor were invaluable to me and this book.

Thanks also to Dana Moreshead from Fishbrain for wrapping it all up in a beautiful package with his striking cover design.

And finally, I give my loving gratitude to my husband Roy, who believed in this book from the beginning and was always there to *keep* me believing.

Contents

Introduction

Do you eat at fast food restaurants? It's okay, a lot of us do. Over 50 percent of Americans, and many people worldwide, eat fast food. We're not going to stop patronizing these establishments. And that's fine. Can you eat a healthy meal at a fast food restaurant? Sure you can. Can you go the other direction? Of course. So it's important to make healthy choices most of the time wherever we eat.

How do you think fast food restaurants stack up to sit-down restaurants, or eating at home? If you think that fast food is always the less healthy diet choice, you're wrong. In fact, the golden arches and the like have often gotten a bad rap, while other dining venues have seemed to skate a bit. This may be one of the reasons why so many Americans are overweight or obese and why this trend is spreading across the globe.

It's important for all of us to take a good hard look at our diets. What did you eat today? Where did you eat it? Was the food nutritious or not so much? How about portion sizes and how the food was prepared? Were you on target there? These are important questions and definitely something to think about.

We all eat food. Every single person on this planet consumes it. It's a basic need and a requirement for life. So, it's a good idea that we all develop a healthy relationship with it.

FAST FOOD VINDICATION

Our dietary preferences vary by country, region, ethnicity, religion, availability, socioeconomic status, individual preference, allergies, and more. Some of us exhibit a passion for food, personally and/or professionally. And the culinary delights that we create for ourselves and others, and purchase from stores and restaurants, run the gamut from simple to extravagant. We buy food from farmers' markets, specialty shops, supermarkets, convenience stores and vending machines. Some of us even grow some of our own food.

There's a lot of information available to us about nutrition and diet. That's fantastic. Some of it's quite good; some of it, not as much. It can be difficult sometimes to determine the best course of action as we navigate the road to nutritious eating and better health. We try many different foods and diets and often look to one thing to hang our hat on, to blame for our too-heavy frames. After all, it's tempting to hold someone or something else responsible for our weighty state of affairs. Fast food restaurants often take the brunt of this blame. From the food that they serve to the jobs that they offer to their expansive growth, these institutions are commonly placed in society's critical crosshairs. Sometimes it's deserved, but not always. We are bombarded with often-conflicting information that can leave us confused and misguided. I aim to change that with this book.

I'm currently a registered dietitian working in the health education department at a major hospital in Southern California. I also teach nutrition to at-risk senior adults as part of a grant program. Prior to this, I spent seven years as a real estate executive at McDonald's Corporation. I'm sure that many of my friends and former co-workers, after finding out that I had left McDonald's in my early forties to go back to school for a master's in nutritional science, would say, "Aha! She was so turned off by the ways of this fast food giant that she left the company to help stop people from eating there." If you think that, you're wrong.

I enjoyed working at McDonald's and think highly of them. They treated me well, and I'm still impressed by their operation and their conduct. I left the company for the reason that so many other people leave good jobs: I was just ready to do something else.

Introduction

As a former insider in the fast food industry, I've seen and heard firsthand the manner in which negative misinformation can affect people and color their opinions. Further, having earned my master's and the credential of registered dietitian (RD), I can speak very specifically and accurately about nutrition and how food, lifestyle, exercise, and other factors impact our health and our waistlines.

What a great many of us haven't yet done is learn how to eat for life, to discern where and how to focus our efforts and to understand how fast food affects our lives. And we should do so. Because fast food is here to stay.

ONE

The Weight of the World Is on Our Shoulders

"Unlike most other nutritionists, I realize that condemning fast food in a culture like ours is a waste of time—it just doesn't work…For one thing, not all fast food is bad. There are quite a few menu items that are highly nutritious and modest in calories."

—Stephen Sinatra, MD, author of *The Fast Food Diet*

My co-worker was going to die because of hamburgers, I thought.

She was dressed in a conservative business suit, standing nose-to-nose with a red-faced man who looked like he wanted to murder her. His hands were clenched so tightly in rage that the skin against his knuckles was paper white. He visibly trembled with anger and anxiety.

We were meeting with area homeowners at a local McDonald's restaurant, on behalf of the corporation, to discuss our plans to open a new location in the neighborhood. And clearly it wasn't going well. The apoplectic man took another step toward my co-worker, but she bravely stood her ground.

I couldn't believe what I was seeing. *She was going to die because of hamburgers.*

My mind flashed back to the other stories I'd heard that should have prepared me for this. A similar situation had occurred at a community meeting that had gotten so ugly that the McDonald's development team members had to hurriedly gather their presentation materials and bolt for their cars. They literally ran. In my mind, I imagined that they were followed by torch-carrying villagers from an old Frankenstein movie.

That's it, I thought as I assessed our current predicament. The angry homeowner and his fellow "villagers" thought we were monsters.

But why? Many of them feared that a new fast food restaurant in the area would bring down property values. Not only is this nowhere near a given in general but we were talking about a location that was on a busy, four-to-six-lane commercial street in Los Angeles, bordered on both sides for miles by all types of businesses, big and small. This included many fast food restaurants. Behind the commercial enterprises were acres of residential real estate, both single and multi-housing, both high end and low income. This state of affairs had existed for many years, likely even before the angry, fist-clenched gentleman standing before us had purchased his home.

The Weight of the World Is on Our Shoulders

It didn't matter. As soon as my co-worker announced our company's proposed intentions, this volatile homeowner leaped to his feet and charged toward her like she was a thief or a murderer who meant him harm.

Luckily we all lived to tell the tale. After a tense minute or so, cooler heads prevailed. Two other attendees were able to pull the homeowner away and calm him down. My co-workers and I then continued our presentation, listened to the man's concerns, and made it out of there safely. Unlike my colleagues before me, we didn't have to dash to our cars.

The experience stuck in my head even after I left McDonald's and became a registered dietitian. Because even though I haven't been employed in the fast food industry in over eight years, it's still a big part of my professional life. I speak about fast food every day when I teach nutrition.

That angry homeowner wasn't the only person I encountered during my McDonald's days who spoke out strongly against the fast food giant's expansion into their area, but he was certainly the scariest. For some, the thought of a McDonald's opening near their homes, even if on a heavily trafficked commercial street, brought out strong and angry emotions. It surprised me every time it happened, but part of me understood. After all these people had heard about the fast food industry, why wouldn't they think that those who worked in it were monsters?

> There were many people who came out ardently in support of proposed McDonald's locations. For them, the addition of a McDonald's (or any national/regional fast food chain) was something to embrace. In fact, one small city in which I secured land for a new McDonald's restaurant was so thrilled that the golden arches were coming to their city, the local high school band marched in celebration on the day of groundbreaking.

Where There's Smoke, Is There Fire?

No question about it, the fast food industry is under attack. There are many who would have you believe that these quick service restaurants are responsible for so much of what's wrong with our world: the obesity epidemic, worldwide cultural homogenization and the proliferation of repetitive, dead-end jobs. These critics maintain that McDonald's, Burger King, Wendy's, Taco Bell, KFC and the like are blights to our landscape and threats to our health. They are indeed not perfect and certainly can and should make some changes (such as more nutritious offerings), but they aren't the horrible and dangerous entities that some would suggest. There's worse out there.

I'm often asked for my thoughts about fast food. These queries usually come from people who have recently read a book, seen a movie, or come across an article with a negative slant on the industry. Or they come from patients sitting across from me, who are looking to incorporate fast food as part of a healthy lifestyle. My response surprises some, but for others it validates what they thought all along. I am firmly in the camp of healthy eating for life. I'm not speaking about diets. I mean *eating for life*. For so many people, this includes fast food. Many of us eat at these restaurants for a variety of reasons, including convenience, cost, and, yes, because we like the food. And that's perfectly acceptable.

There are definitely things about the fast food industry that I'm not crazy about. From a health perspective, it's true that their menus are loaded with high-fat, high-calorie items, like the Carl's Jr. Six Dollar Burger, the McDonald's McFlurry (even the smoothies are high in calories), Wendy's Double and Triple burgers, Burger King's double and triple burgers, Taco Bell's Grilled Stuft Burrito and KFC's Double Down sandwich (a piece of meat between two pieces of fried chicken masquerading as a bun), to name a few. This list could certainly be expanded to quite a long one. Plus, the sodium content of many of their menu items is off the charts. But while this isn't good news, it's not unique to fast food. We need to open our eyes to this.

The Weight of the World Is on Our Shoulders

And yet there's a positive trend in evidence as more and more of the fast food establishments are offering better nutritional alternatives to their less healthy fare. Most of their menus now contain lighter choices, such as garden burgers, grilled chicken sandwiches, salads, apple slices, carrot sticks, baked potatoes and fruit and yogurt parfaits. And a special mention must be made of the turkey burgers introduced by Carl's Jr. that were developed in conjunction with the staff of *Men's Health/Eat This Not That*. This is a positive development, in which publications devoted to health and better eating have collaborated with a fast food restaurant for the good of its customers. But be warned that even a healthier protein choice like a turkey burger over a beef patty can be made into a less healthy sandwich. So make good choices on what you put on and next to that burger.

So, armed with a bit of knowledge (and self-discipline), it isn't so difficult to incorporate nutritious fast food items into a healthy lifestyle. It's important to be aware, to be knowledgeable and to accept responsibility for our own actions. This is sometimes easier said than done, but in many ways our health is ours to make or break. But a good number of us tend to forget that we hold most of the cards. I help my patients and clients understand this and provide them with the knowledge that they need to navigate the sometimes confusing and tempting world of food and eating. I'll also help you, my readers, do this in the later chapters of this book.

The Buck Stops Here

But let's not forget we are human. Taking responsibility for our own actions can be difficult. Avoiding eating that piece of cake, ignoring the salt shaker, or taking a walk around the block can seem impossible. Many of us may even be in denial and not facing what's right in front of us. We've all been there. Sometimes we just want to blame someone else for something that mostly rests on our own shoulders.

FAST FOOD VINDICATION

In recent years, there have been some high-profile critics of the fast food industry, including Eric Schlosser (author of the best-selling book *Fast Food Nation*), Morgan Spurlock (writer/director of the documentary *Super Size Me*) and several physician and community groups. Important information can be garnered from all of these sources. While I applaud them for making dietary and other important issues a part of the national dialogue, I don't agree with all of their messages. On the subject of healthy eating and fast food, I have a different take.

With respect to the obesity epidemic, I don't look at fast food as the only culprit. We need to take a wider, more objective look at all that we eat, where we consume it and how much we move. We must take responsibility for our own choices and actions, but that can be a tall order. And we need to come up with realistic solutions to help us make appropriate changes.

Recently, several overweight/obese people have sued fast food chains for damages related to their weight gains. These people held the restaurants, not themselves, responsible for their excess pounds. It appears they didn't feel that they personally had much to do with it. This is worrisome not only for them but for the many others out there who may feel just like these plaintiffs did. Yes, it would be so much easier if we could look at others as the cause for our weight gain. Those reliant on someone to buy and/or prepare their food (such as children or people with health issues who need assistance), have a bit of an argument here, but outside of this, most of the rest of us don't.

At the hospital where I work, we have a fantastic curriculum for teaching our diabetes classes. One part of it brings home the point of personal responsibility: In big bold letters in the middle of the page is the word "YOU," with spokes jutting out to various things we should do to manage the condition, such as education, activity/exercise and meal planning. The point is to illustrate that while others can assist us, most of the burden of taking care of ourselves lies nowhere else but with us. My co-workers and I tell our patients that 90 percent of their own care comes from them. Ten percent comes from others, like the health care team. This concept applies to most of us for many things, including the weight that we carry on our frames. Laying blame at others' doorsteps just doesn't cut it. Suing a fast food restaurant, or any other restaurant for that matter, focuses too much of the blame on one of the spokes, not on "YOU," the true bull's-eye.

We're the quarterbacks here. And while we typically don't have control over others, we usually can manage ourselves. In most cases, we choose our food, the amount we eat, the frequency of our overeating and our physical activity levels. I've been in many a fast food restaurant in my time, and I can't remember one of them telling me what I would eat and force-feeding me food against my will. Now, there could be many other issues at play with regard to how we eat, such as lack of self-control, mental and/or physical issues and/or a limited knowledge of nutrition. All of these are real and understandable. However, they're still our personal responsibilities. Certainly they should be addressed. Help is out there. It isn't always easy, so many of us go kicking and screaming into change. But that doesn't mean it's someone else's fault.

Of the various lawsuits brought against fast food establishments alleging that they were the cause of the plaintiff's obesity and/or health-related issues, some were dropped. Others went in favor of the defendants, the fast food corporations. Congress eventually passed legislation to prevent frivolous lawsuits of this type from clogging the judicial system.

Our choices are our own. We can make wise decisions or not. We can also help shape what the market offers us. It's called supply and demand. Many of us buy things that cause others to then turn around and blame the business that responds and offers the items. Conflicting viewpoints are normal. In addition, when a business sells a product that not enough people buy, it's typically not fiscally viable for the company to continue to sell that product. This happens all the time, including in the fast food industry.

In the mid-1990s, Taco Bell offered a light menu, and I absolutely adored the fat-free bean burrito, which was a healthier choice than many of the other menu items that were then offered. I had one for lunch every Saturday for about a year. I looked forward to it all week long. It was that good.

One Saturday, I cheerfully entered the drive-thru at my neighborhood Taco Bell, mouth watering in anticipation. I drove up to the order point and cheerfully asked for one fat-free bean burrito. "I'm sorry, ma'am," replied the voice from the speaker. "We don't have that anymore. Can I get you something else?" I couldn't believe my ears, and it wasn't because he had called me ma'am. Unfortunately, Taco Bell had discontinued its light menu, probably due to sales expectations not being met. They had built it, but not enough had come.

When asked what else I might want instead of the defunct fat-free bean burrito, I was stymied. The reality at the time was that there weren't many healthier choices left at this restaurant after the removal of the light fare menu. I did make a choice, though. I ordered nothing. Just because they offered it didn't mean that I should, or would, eat it.

Happily, perhaps due to a change in customer demand, Taco Bell introduced its fresco menu with lighter choices many years later. Most of the other fast food chains offer healthier items as well. It's up to the consumer, you and me, to keep these items on the menu by buying them. It's certainly okay to have a hamburger and french fries from time to time, and many of us do just that. These items aren't likely to disappear anytime soon. But we need to buy the healthier choices if we want them to be there for us.

The danger of heaping blame on the fast food industry, especially to the exclusion of other causes, is that it may obscure other threats—and solutions. There's a serious obesity epidemic in the United States and it's a growing problem throughout the world. Lifestyle diseases such as type 2 diabetes are dangerously on the rise. Pointing a finger at fast food as the major, if not sole, contributor to this state of affairs minimizes other factors including: larger portion sizes at sit-down restaurants; decreased or non-existent physical activity; increased caloric intake from snacks, sodas and energy drinks; and the content and size of foods prepared at home. It's indeed a dangerous path to take and one that does not solve the problem at hand.

And again, I must stress that the most important factor is "us." We must ask the question, are we actively looking for ways to help ourselves? We can't all answer in the affirmative. *USA Today* recently reported on the results of an online survey for the International Food Information Council (IFIC) Foundation. The purpose was to help ascertain how Americans were monitoring their caloric intakes. It turns out that among the respondents, only a very small number of people (nine percent) correctly estimated the amount of calories they should consume in one day. More concerning is that only nine percent even kept track of the calories they actually ate daily. A variety of reasons were given for this: no interest, knowledge or focus; an uncertainty that calories are that important to track; and the difficulty of keeping tabs on caloric intake. These reasons apply not only to fast food venues but to the entire scope of our daily eating lives.

We would be much better served by looking at the bigger and truer picture. While some actually seek to ban new fast food restaurants in their cities, this doesn't solve anything except taking away one of the fundamental rights of Americans: freedom of choice. It's much more effective to educate ourselves so that when we do eat fast food, or any kind of food at any type of venue, we'll be equipped to make healthier meal choices.

From Building Restaurants to Fostering Good Health

I went to school with many exceptional and intelligent people who have gone on to become successful RDs, making a positive impact on the health of people of all ages. I'd have the utmost confidence in putting my and my loved ones' nutritional health in their hands. But during several years' worth of class discussions, I became a bit concerned by some of my fellow students' narrow—indeed, almost militant—views on how America, and the world, should eat. One classmate felt that everyone should cook all of their own meals, never eating out at any restaurant of any type. This would definitely not work for me and my husband and the majority of my friends and family. Some felt that getting people to totally abandon fast food would solve most of society's nutritional problems. Others were big proponents of all-organic products and growing most of our own food. What I wouldn't give to have that kind of time and focus! These academic-based theories all have some merit but aren't realistic for most of us. Moderation and balance is often an easier and more practical way to go.

As is true of many college students, regardless of age, sometimes our ideas change as we get out into the real world. One of my classmates was very big on making major changes to school lunches, abolishing all unhealthy offerings. Lots of fruits and vegetables, preferably organic, lean proteins and whole grains, with no junk food or typical "kid" foods, was her dream. She was quite adamant about it, and in concept it's a wonderful idea. But I never thought it was realistic. Kids can be challenging, and food is one of those areas where many children and adolescents dig in their heels.

I was told during one of the internships required for my license that plate waste studies had shown that often the whole fruit on the school lunch tray ended up in the trash—still whole. Not good, but not a surprise to me. In the case of my classmate who felt strongly about radically changing the school cafeteria, she followed her interest and took a job as a dietitian at a high school in an upscale city in Los Angeles County. She graduated a year before I did and came back afterward to speak to my class about her work experience. She informed everyone that once she left the confines of school and entered the "real world," she realized her vision wasn't so easy to implement. School cafeterias typically have to make money, or at least not lose money, so it's important that they offer what the students will buy. In the case of the high school where my classmate worked, what they wanted was pizza and fries, two items she was loathe to offer. Since she didn't want to lose money, she ended up selling them. That was practical. But she took it a step further and made sure that the pizza had low-fat cheese and vegetables and that the fries were baked. That was smart.

The Weight of the World Is on Our Shoulders

It's a lesson that many dietitians have learned. Reinventing the wheel won't be embraced by most of us. Learning to lighten up even foods such as pizza and fries may be more palatable (pun intended) for many.

> In the 2012 HBO documentary series *The Weight of the Nation,* a very amazing group of school kids in a group called the Rethinkers was showcased. Formed in 2006 with just 20 Louisiana middle-school kids, the group aimed to "give a voice in rebuilding schools" after Hurricane Katrina. Its first mission was to improve meals in schools. And they had some success. In May 2011, the Rethinkers convinced Aramark, the company providing the school's meals, to serve locally- grown produce a minimum of two days per school week.
>
> At this writing, the Rethink program has 100 student members and ten adult staffers. For more information on their fantastic effort, visit therethinkers.com.

> A school in Chicago banned bag lunches, requiring its students to eat the school provided lunch. The principal said that she instituted this policy because the students "were bringing junk food to the school."

After I graduated and moved into the health care field, I found myself working with patients on a wide range of nutritional issues. A substantial part of my job is teaching classes on diabetes, high cholesterol (hyperlipidemia), hypertension (high blood pressure), healthy eating and weight management.

FAST FOOD VINDICATION

I've seen thousands of patients and many of them are quite knowledgeable and proactive in managing their own health. It's wonderful to see. There are others who are motivated and would like to do better but don't yet have all of the knowledge and skills to accomplish this goal. They need help. This is a large group, and I would hazard to guess that there are a lot of other people out there who would also like more information so that they can better help themselves.

And it's out there. One of the many tools at our disposal is the nutrition information for some sit-down and fast food restaurants. This data enables us to make better choices and analyze the different types of restaurant meal offerings. It also provides a way to see how menu items at different restaurants stack up. In comparing the Chili's Grill & Bar Classic Bacon Burger with Burger King's Smoked Bacon and Cheddar Angus burger, the Burger King sandwich—while still too high in calories, fat and sodium—comes out on top. The Chili's burger contains 1,080 calories, 71 g of fat and 1,660 mg of sodium, while the BK burger has 674 calories, 38 g of fat and 835 mg of sodium. You might be shocked to discover that the Chili's burger is the worse choice and that there are scores of other higher-calorie and higher-fat options at a lot of other sit-down restaurants. The portions are typically too big and there are more choices for expanding the meal, such as including an appetizer in the order.

In addition, most sit-down restaurants drop a bread or chip basket in the middle of the table and keep it full. For free! This can be a major pitfall. The bread basket is not our friend. We might eat more calories out of it than we should in the whole meal, or even the whole day. Many of us don't give this part of the meal much thought. My husband is one. He recently ate three baskets of tortilla chips at our local Mexican restaurant. I couldn't believe my eyes. He, like most of us, should make a few healthy changes in his diet.

Beverages can also be another downfall. Quite a few of us don't think about the calories in our drinks, but many of our liquid refreshments are jam-packed with them. And don't get me started on the salads. At sit-down restaurants, they're not always the healthy fare we tend to think they are. If we order fried chicken in our fast food salads, they can be a problem too. I will discuss all of this later on.

Recently, my hospital's health education department prepared a presentation for the physicians. It included a quiz about the calorie content of entrées at sit-down restaurants. A good number of the MDs, and even some of the dietitians in our department, were quite surprised by the hefty numbers of calories they contained.

While many see fast food as unhealthy, a lot of us will go to sit-down restaurants and eat far more calories, carbohydrate, sodium and fat than we would at the Burger Kings and KFCs of the world. The portion sizes, ingredients and methods of preparation at so many sit-down restaurants, including those that quite a few would label as "healthy," can be incredibly large and loaded with many bad things for us. We can also overeat and make less healthy choices at home and other places where we eat.

But criticism of the fast food industry goes beyond the menu items, and here the negative claims may be overstated as well. And because the media don't often highlight its positive aspects, many don't know about the significant contributions the industry makes worldwide. From its small beginnings to the global entities of today, the fast food industry's history is indeed an amazing story. An inside look—from its start, to the food it offers, the jobs it provides, its philanthropic efforts and its significance to the world economy—will open a few eyes. By the time you finish this book, you'll not only know more of the truth about the fast food industry, you'll also have the tools you need to make better food choices, whether at fast food restaurants, sit-down restaurants or at home.

FAST FOOD VINDICATION

Fast food isn't the enemy. It's an integral part of the American lifestyle, and it now has roots in many other countries around the world. It won't simply disappear from our landscape. Nor should it. Instead we should recognize the industry for its contributions to society and learn how to incorporate its products into a healthy lifestyle. Sensible eating can include fast food. The time has come to educate America, and the world, about how to best eat for life. The time has come for fast food vindication.

Two

The Fattening of America
...and the World

"People are responsible for what they eat, not restaurants."

**—Merab Morgan, woman who lost weight on a
McDonald's food-only diet**

America is fat. We're the land of excess, both good and bad. We eat too much, sit too much and don't exercise enough. We often think bigger is better, and this includes the portion sizes of our foods. We typically serve our meals on bigger plates than we should. At some sit-down restaurants, they're as large as platters. And we fill these plates to the edge, often with unhealthy items. Portion sizes have grown over the years, and inevitably, *we've* gotten bigger.

I embarrass my husband to no end because I often bring a scale, measuring cups and measuring spoons with me when we go out to eat. I'm sure he's considered sitting at a separate table. I bring these kitchen gadgets because I'm curious about how much food we're being served. And let me tell you, it's absolutely jaw-dropping.

Some of the worst offenders that come to mind include my favorite Italian restaurants in and around Los Angeles, both chain and mom-and-pop. Most of these establishments tend to give 4 to 8 servings of pasta in *one* entrée. And the heaps of dressing, avocado and cheese piled on the salads fill the bowls to the cavernous brim.

> Don't let folded items like burritos fool you. Recently my husband and I went to our favorite local Mexican restaurant. My burrito-loving spouse ordered just that. It looked quite large in its prepared state, so I asked him to unfold it before eating it. He nicely complied. The tortilla practically could've been used as a tablecloth. It was that big. It could have fed two to three people.

Approximately two-thirds of adults 20 and older in America are overweight or obese. And it's recently been projected that 42 percent of Americans could be obese by the year 2030. There's no question that we're in the midst of an alarming epidemic. Both overweight and obesity rates are at an all-time high in the United States.

> A U.S. Center for Disease Control and Prevention analysis of a 2010 survey revealed that Colorado is the only state in America with an obesity rate less than 20 percent. And twelve states' rates are a whopping 30 percent or more.

But America isn't the only country experiencing this problem. This is a worldwide concern. Around the globe in 2008, about one male in ten was obese, as was one in seven females. And it's an upward trajectory with the World Health Organization predicting that there will be more than 2 billion overweight people around the world by 2015. You read it correctly...*2 billion.* Of those, 700 million will be considered to be obese.

Adult *Obese* Populations by Country	
Naru	78.5%
Tonga	56.0%
Saudi Arabia	35.6%
United Arab Emirates	33.7%
United States	32.2%
Bahrain	28.9%
Kuwait	28.8%
Seychelles	25.1%
United Kingdom	24.2%

So how did we get here and what does it all mean? Who's overweight? Is it you? Is it me? And what exactly does being overweight or obese mean? The important thing to know is that carrying around an excess amount of pounds on our frames can cause a host of health problems. Too much body weight goes hand in hand with many disease states. They love each other, are husband and wife, are best friends for life. So it's imperative that we all strive to maintain a healthy weight by eating a balanced, nutritious diet and engaging in physical activity on a regular basis.

The topic of weight is often at the forefront in newspapers and magazines, and many news programs regularly feature health segments discussing food intake. This is all great. But it doesn't always sink into the brains of those of us who need it. Does every overweight person know, in fact, that they are overweight? For the very obese, they likely do. But many of us are walking around today who have no idea that we are indeed overweight. And very few of us are immune. Overweight and obesity in adults of both genders have increased over the years in all ethnic groups, ages and education levels.

Are You Overweight or Obese?

One indicator, body mass index (BMI), takes our weight in pounds and divides it by height in inches squared. This number is then multiplied by 703.

For example, a woman who is 5'4" (64 inches) tall and weighs 150 pounds would divide 150 by 4,096 (64 x 64, height in inches squared). The number obtained, 0.037, would then be multiplied by 703. This woman has a BMI of 25.7.

There are also BMI calculators online.

BMI RANGES
18.5 to 24.9 is healthy
25 to 29.9 is overweight
30 and over is obese

Therefore, the above example of the woman with a 25.7 BMI means she would be categorized as overweight.

Waist Circumference

Another important measurement is waist circumference (WC). A female with a WC greater than 35" and a male with a WC greater than 40" with a BMI in the overweight to obese range may have an increased risk for high cholesterol, hypertension, heart disease and type 2 diabetes. WC is also helpful for a person who has more muscle mass, like an athlete, whose bulk may cause him or her to have a BMI of 25 or over.

Obesity and Disease

When we discuss the consequences of the obesity epidemic, we're not just talking about the unhappiness some of us feel in having to buy the next size jeans or the reluctance to take off our cover-ups at the beach. I don't know about you, but I'm reluctant to take off my cover-up at *any* weight. All kidding aside, the ramifications of the obesity epidemic are much more serious than physical appearance, because they can lead to a myriad of problems and diseases.

HEALTH ISSUES ASSOCIATED WITH OVERWEIGHT/OBESITY		
Diabetes	Hypertension	Stroke
Heart Disease	High Cholesterol	Osteoarthritis
Gallbladder Disease	Sleep Apnea	Some Cancers
Kidney Disease	Menstrual Irregularities	Pregnancy Complications
Incontinence	Depression	Increased Surgical Risk

As obesity levels rise, so do death rates. People who are obese have a greater risk (10 to 50 percent) of death from all causes. Most of the increased risk is due to cardiovascular disease. Obesity causes approximately 112,000 additional deaths in the United States each year. My father was one casualty. He was overweight and suffered from several lifestyle diseases. He had diabetes, hypertension, heart disease, high cholesterol and cancer. And I have no doubt that his weight was a key contributor to some of these conditions, which led to his death at the young age of 68.

> Because of my family history of heart disease and high cholesterol, I haven't eaten red meat in over 35 years. I don't even remember what it tastes like. And my cholesterol is much the better for it.

And let's not overlook what being obese does to our pocketbooks. Carrying too much weight on our frames can cost us money. A study by the George Washington University School of Public Health found that it costs obese men in the United States close to $2,700 and obese American women almost $4,900 to carry that extra weight each year. I don't know about you, but I'd rather put that money to a different use.

I frequently ask my patients to visualize a seesaw with a person standing over each end, but neither one has yet sat down. This is how we want everything in our bodies to be, balanced and within recommended ranges. When we do something that doesn't keep within healthy parameters, such as carry too much weight on our frames, someone sits down on the seesaw and we tilt. Tilting opens us up for complications and puts us at increased risk for certain diseases.

> According to the American Diabetes Association, even if the "prevalence of obesity" stabilizes through 2030, the number of diabetes cases will more than double those in 2007.

A recent study of close to 5,000 adults 18 and older (average age of 44) found that engaging in certain bad habits, such as inactivity, poor diet, drinking too much alcohol and smoking, can age you by *12 years*. I don't know how you feel about that, but for me my time already moves by fast enough. I'm not looking to prematurely age myself. The good news is that if we've "tilted" by carrying too much weight on our frames, or by having one or more of the above unhealthy behaviors, we can make necessary changes and get that imaginary person on that seesaw to stand up, getting us back to—or much closer to—that nice straight line.

The Young Are Not Immune

Unfortunately, weight problems aren't limited to the adult population. The number one health issue facing children and adolescents in the United States today is obesity. Approximately one in three American children and adolescents is overweight or obese. The CDC reports that about 17 percent of those aged 2 to 19 in the U.S. are obese. Worldwide, approximately 20 million children under the age of 5 were considered to be obese in 2005. An overweight child is at risk for many of the same health problems that threaten adults, including heart disease, hypertension, and high cholesterol.

Alarmingly, children are also developing what was once called adult-onset diabetes. Currently labeled type 2 diabetes, this disease now afflicts even young children. Also, overweight adolescents have a 70 percent chance of becoming an overweight or obese adult. But the effects aren't just physical. Often these children also face issues such as depression, poor self-esteem and social discrimination.

In recent years, there's been an increase in news stories about specific children who are alarmingly obese. And while the United States currently appears to have the dubious distinction of having the most overweight or obese children and adolescents (approximately 37 percent), other countries seem to be making a concerted effort to capture that top spot. According to a recent *Time* magazine article, statistics reported at the European Congress on Obesity showed that over 20 percent of Europeans between 5 and 17 were either overweight or obese. Childhood obesity is also on the rise in the Middle East, North Africa and Asia. Sadly, there are too many stories to tell, but the following provides the gist:

In March 2011, a 3-year-old boy in China, Lu Hao, weighed 132 pounds. He was so heavy that his mother could no longer pick him up. At the time, Hao's parents said he could eat three large bowls of rice in one meal, more than either his mother or father consumed. While they were trying to regulate what he ate, Hao's mother said, "We have to let him be [because] if we don't feed him he will cry non-stop." Not surprisingly, Hao doesn't like to walk.

Then there's the case of the 5-foot tall, 8-year-old boy from England who in 2007 weighed 218 pounds, over three times what the average boy weighs at that age. By the time he was 2, he weighed so much that his mother couldn't lift him. She said he "eats double or triple" the amount of food that he should and that he "steals and hides food."

Health agencies worked with the boy's mother to determine if he should be taken into protective care, citing that while they were working with the family, there were many missed appointments with nutritionists, social workers and nurses. Ultimately, the mother was permitted to retain custody of her son. An unnamed source said, "Child abuse is not just about hitting your children or sexually abusing them; it is also about neglect."

Dr. Colin Waine, then director of the National Obesity Forum in Nottingham, England, said the boy's lifestyle was "extremely dangerous" and that he was "at risk for developing diabetes in his early teens...[and] cardiovascular and nervous system problems in his 20s." Waine added, "He's really at risk of dying by the time he's 30." Unfortunately, he isn't the only child in Britain whose weight is concerning. In 2008, seven children were placed in the care of social services because they were morbidly obese.

> More recently, the walls of 19-year-old Georgia Davis's home had to be cut open to remove her from the structure. At approximately 882 pounds, she was known as Britain's heaviest teenager. In the young woman's words, "Some people choose heroin but I've chosen food and it's killing me." It appears that most of her weight came not from fast food, but from food prepared at home. She spoke of eating two entire loaves worth of sandwiches filled with jam, cheese or meat every day. Her daily food intake also included five bags of cheese and onion crisps, two packages of chocolate bourbon candy, sponge cake, chocolate cake, plus a dinner of four sausages and mashed potatoes with baked beans.

Back in America, 14-year-old South Carolinian Alexander Draper weighed 555 pounds in 2009. At this weight, he'd have been at risk for many lifestyle-related diseases and even premature death. His mother, Jerri Gray, went on the run with him after failing to keep medical appointments made by the Department of Social Services. Coupled with Draper's continued weight gain, this led to her losing custody of Alexander. She was arrested and charged with child neglect and custodial interference. Alexander was placed in foster care. This case sparked debate about whether child obesity is abuse. After all, was Gray able to control everything that her son ate?

A recent study by Canadian researchers compared 63 obese kids to 55 children who were at a healthy weight. The results showed that the arteries of the obese children were prematurely aging. In particular, the obese kid's aortas were stiff. In response to the study, Dr. Beth Abramson, spokesperson for the Heart and Stroke Foundation, reported: "Our kids are at risk. Poor nutrition and inactivity are threatening their health and well-being. We must rethink the lifestyle standards we have accepted as a society to protect the future health of our kids."

I meet one-on-one and teach classes with children/adolescents of all ages and their parents. There are many who are proactive and I applaud their efforts. But on every class roster or individual consult appointment, there are always cancellations and no-shows. I understand that life sometimes gets in the way of us being able to make every appointment. And I get it, you teens, it's not the most fun thing in the world to go to a weight management class. But it can definitely be worthwhile. If it prompts healthy change, no matter how small, it's worth it.

Being overweight or obese can be quite detrimental to our health at any age. Four of the top ten causes of death in America (diabetes, cancer, stroke and heart disease) can be related to diet and lifestyle. Other conditions, such as hypertension, high cholesterol, osteoporosis and obesity, may also be attributed in part to poor diet practices. It's never too early in life to start eating healthier to help ward off these conditions.

Here's a sobering proposition: the latest generation born in the United States may be the first to have a shorter life span than the one that came before.

THREE

The Blame Game

"Obesity is a bad problem, but to single out one component of the diets as a silver bullet to fix it is fantasy."

—Dr. James Rippe, cardiologist

Americans love a hero. We enjoy watching a lone figure battle the all-powerful enemy, the villain who is causing so many of the world's ills. Fast food has certainly played the role of the malefactor. Morgan Spurlock (*Super Size Me*) and Eric Schlosser (*Fast Food Nation*) could be considered pioneers in taking hard looks at the fast food industry. They took the rather uncompromising position that fast food is bad for our health and our society and should be avoided, if not obliterated even from the world.

There are certainly components of their messages that should be heeded. The significance of their contribution and their impact can't be overstated. They got us thinking about important topics, and we still talk about them today.

For sure, fast food restaurants have their share of less-healthy food. But critics often overlook the fact that they also offer healthier items as well. And too little is said about the other places where we eat—full-service, sit-down establishments that offer many less-healthy menu items, as well as schools, vending machines, supermarkets, convenience stores and our homes. It's crucial that we're aware of this, and too many of us aren't.

The Spurlock Regimen

For the film *Super Size Me*, Morgan Spurlock came up with an attention-getting idea: for thirty days, he ate all of his meals at McDonald's restaurants while movie cameras tracked his progress. His weight and health were monitored to see how things changed while on the McDonald's-only diet. It was pretty ingenious and interesting to see. He set parameters, such as whenever asked by the counter person if he would like to supersize his meal to a larger-size french fries and beverage, he did so, which happened nine times over the 30-day period. He also attempted to cut his physical activity to 2.5 miles a day, or 5,000 steps, although he averaged about three miles a day prior to filming. Spurlock informed us that most Americans at the time walked approximately 1.5 miles a day.

At the outset, a dietitian told Spurlock that he required approximately 2,500 calories a day to maintain his body weight. For the most part, Spurlock doubled that amount in the food he chose from the McDonald's menus. Therefore he was eating approximately 5,000 calories a day.

Spurlock's criteria required him to have every menu item at least once during the 30 days. He seemed to favor higher-calorie foods, such as the Double Quarter Pounder with Cheese Extra Value Meal (which comes with fries and a drink), milkshakes, regular Cokes and Big Macs. Does this sound familiar to any of you? He appeared to limit lighter items. This created a high-calorie/high-fat intake that demonstrated how unhealthy choices can lead to excess. By examining his choices, we can see how better decisions can be made.

Spurlock could have chosen many McDonald's food items that are much lower in calories, fat and cholesterol. You and I can do that as well. For breakfast, instead of ordering the Egg McMuffin Extra Value meal for breakfast, he could've ordered an English muffin with grape jelly (195 calories—or, better yet, dry for less calories), a snack size parfait with granola (160 calories—or without the granola for fewer calories), and black coffee with artificial sweetener (0 calories), for a total of 355 calories. Or he could have just had the Egg McMuffin on its own, which would have cost him just 300 calories. Today, you could add Apple Slices, which is a good choice that has only 15 calories. Oatmeal is also offered now, but monitor the portion size and the toppings.

For lunch or dinner, instead of a Double Quarter Pounder Extra Value Meal, Spurlock could've ordered a grilled chicken sandwich without mayonnaise (350 calories), with a side salad with low-fat Italian dressing (80 calories) and iced tea with artificial sweetener (0 calories) for a total of 450 calories. With regard to his beverage of choice, Spurlock often seemed to order regular Coca-Cola, which has a lot of sugar and calories, but he could have opted for the Diet Coke, which has 0 calories. Or how about water? It's the gold standard. I could go on and on, but I'm sure you get the point.

I'm from Atlanta, which is a Coca-Cola town. Go Coke! I have a friend who's a pretty healthy eater and physically active, but even so, he'd started to gain weight. He was stymied about what to do to reverse this trend and asked for my advice. I happened to know that he was drinking regular Cokes. I asked how many he was drinking each day. He replied that he was having four regular Cokes a day, which likely meant six! One 12-ounce Coke has 140 calories. The 20-ounce version has 240 calories. I suggested that at the very least he switch to Diet Coke. Drinking water instead would be even better. He went with Diet Coke and made no other changes. Guess what? You go it! He lost the weight that he'd gained.

What about healthier choices at fast food restaurants? In *Don't Eat This Book,* Spurlock writes that when filming *Super Size Me,* he made it a point to order a salad every ten meals. Is this indicative of the average fast food consumer?

Let's take a look at salads. They've been rising in popularity at fast food restaurants. Between 2003 and 2006, McDonald's sold 500 million of them, for a total of over $2 billion. In 2007, Technomic Information Services, which monitors the fast food industry, found that salads at fast food venues were exhibiting strong growth and "consumers were more likely to consider quick-service [fast food] ahead of quick-casual [sit-down], especially at lunch."

In a 2010 interview, McDonald's spokesperson Danya Proud said the fast food giant is one of the largest sellers of salads in the United States, while sales of the company's Apple Dippers were "tremendous."

Outside of his film, Spurlock does seem to favor healthier food. If he found himself at McDonald's for reasons other than his documentary, he might have made more balanced, sensible choices such as salads. We have the opportunity to do this as well. While the offerings of lighter menu items at McDonald's and other fast food restaurants have increased, it's true that many people choose the less nutritious menu items on a regular basis. That's why it's important to know how to integrate fast food into a healthy way of life.

Few McDonald's customers (or those of other fast food restaurants) eat the way that Spurlock does in his documentary. The percentage of the U.S. population who eat all three of their meals every day at McDonald's is tiny, even for periods much shorter than Spurlock's 30 days. In fact, several studies have shown that while fast food consumption in the United States is high, the typical customer doesn't eat it nearly as frequently as Spurlock does in his documentary.

One University of Minnesota study followed 3,031 Caucasian and African American adults aged 18 to 30. Results showed that men ate at fast food restaurants more often than women, as did African Americans over Caucasians. In 2000 to 2001, African American men visited fast food restaurants 2.3 times per week on average. Caucasian women made 1.3 visits per week. That's nowhere close to eating three meals a day, seven days a week, I'm happy to say. That would simply be too much.

A comparison of two U.S. Department of Agriculture (USDA) studies that surveyed what 9,872 adults 20 and older ate on two different days found that 5,861 of the participants did not eat fast food on *either* of the two days. That's over half of the participants. Of the 2,623 who consumed fast food on one of the day's studies, only 838 of these had it on both days. And in *Fast Food Nation*, Eric Schlosser reports that the average American eats approximately three hamburgers and four orders of french fries each week. While that's arguably too much, it's not anywhere close to what Spurlock gobbled down in *Super Size Me*. This is good.

FAST FOOD VINDICATION

So, while fast food consumption in the United States and world-wide is high, studies suggest that most people in the United States don't even eat one meal per day, every day of the week, at a fast food restaurant. More recent data shows that over 50 percent of adults dine outside the home three or more times per week.

> A survey of over 210,000 people found that 96 percent of adults in the U.S. eat out at a restaurant at least one time in a typical month. In the average 30 day time frame, 91 percent eat at a fast food restaurant and 84 percent dine at a sit-down establishment.

One-third of calories consumed in America come from restaurant food of all types. That's significant, but we need to examine the other areas from which our calories come. Where do we get the rest? Certainly home is one of the most important places. A recent Marist Poll found that 58 percent of Americans ate dinner at home at least six times per week.

> There are indeed those folks who eat very frequently at fast food restaurants. McDonald's has quite the loyal customer in Wisconsinite Don Gorske. He recently ate his 25,000[th] Big Mac. The 59-year-old has been eating, on average, two of these sandwiches every day. He says, "I plan on eating Big Macs until I die. I have no intention of changing. It's my favorite food. Nothing has changed in 39 years. I look forward to it every day." He claims his health is good and that his cholesterol level is low. Perhaps he's just one of those lucky people with good genes! Nevertheless, this isn't something that I would recommend.

On the subject of cholesterol, let's take another look at Spurlock and *Super Size Me*. Over the course of the film's thirty-day period, Spurlock gained 24.5 pounds. His total cholesterol increased from 168 mg/dL to 230 mg/dL, which is well above the recommended level of less than 200 mg/dL. In addition, his liver levels increased to a very unhealthy degree, although at the end of the period they showed signs of improvement.

None of this is shocking. The sheer calorie count and quality of his diet definitely impacted him. One pound equals 3,500 calories. So with a daily consumption of 5,000 calories and a dietitian telling him 2,500 calories was his maintenance level, Spurlock ingested something like 2,500 excess calories *every day*. This equates to a five pound weight gain each week. Who wants that?

But it doesn't stop there. As noted before, Spurlock also reduced his activity level. At the beginning of *Super Size Me*, we're told that he walks to his office, which is over one mile away from his apartment. We're left to assume that he walks much more than just the several-mile round trip he takes to and from work. But for the duration of his thirty-day film, he drastically cuts his physical activity, resulting in even more weight gain. He eats twice the number of calories he should in a day and significantly decreases his physical activity. So it stands to reason that he suffered because of it. Most of us would as well.

There's no great mystery to weight gain. If calories consumed exceed calories expended, we will gain weight. That's all there is to it. Calories that aren't used are stored as fat in the body. Exercise can help a person lose or maintain weight by burning these excess calories.

In 2005, the National Institutes of Health reported the results of a ten-year observational study that found that girls who weren't active during adolescence gained on average between 10 to 15 more pounds than girls who were active. In an eight-month study by Duke University Medical Center, 120 sedentary and overweight adults were monitored. They were placed into four groups. Three of the groups engaged in various levels of exercise. One group didn't exercise at all.

The participants were all asked to make no changes in their normal dietary intake, so, unlike Spurlock, they didn't add any additional calories. The participants who exercised saw a *decrease* in their waist circumferences. The non-exercisers saw a 0.8-inch *increase*. Other studies have pointed to exercise as a means to improved body weight maintenance.

Exercise is good for us; it helps us manage our weight. It also increases our general level of fitness and can lower the risk of certain diseases. In addition, physical activity can help reduce anxiety and depression, and improve self-esteem.

Through scenes with his doctors, Spurlock makes the point that being overweight is harmful to our health. He showed us that his weight, cholesterol and other lab values were negatively impacted due to his overeating, lack of exercise and excessive weight gain.

Many critics assailed Spurlock's tactics, and he himself admits (in his 2005 bestseller, *Don't Eat This Book*) that *Super Size Me* was "a stunt" but a "stunt with a very serious message behind it." Gorging on unhealthy foods to the point that you harm yourself is definitely serious, as is America's (and the world's) obesity epidemic. Spurlock was definitely spot-on in tackling the issue, and many listened. But I'm not sure everyone learned. What exactly was the long-term impact? Did it affect the eating habits of those who ate at fast food restaurants? Did it affect McDonald's?

In an interview with Danya Proud of McDonald's Corporation, I asked just that question. According to Proud, sales actually *increased* after *Super Size Me* debuted. McDonald's served 2 million more customers the year the film came out than they had the year before. People still frequented McDonald's in large numbers. I also asked Proud to weigh in on the common perception that McDonald's eliminated its "supersizing" option because of Spurlock's film. Her answer was a swift and adamant "no." She said that change was already in the works before the film—and, as is true of most large corporations, the wheels turn slowly and change is slow to come. An independent conversation with a senior vice president of McDonald's Corporation corroborated this.

And unfortunately, we know Spurlock's film didn't help to reverse the growing size of many of our girths. It's difficult for many of us to change. While *Super Size Me* created awareness, it didn't provide us with the building blocks for change.

Supersize vs. Undersize

In response to *Super Size Me*, several people countered the film's premise by losing weight on McDonald's-only diets. In 2005, Merab Morgan ate every meal at McDonald's for 90 days. At the beginning of the diet, she weighed 227 pounds. In contrast to Spurlock's overindulging, Morgan consulted nutrition information from the McDonald's website and devised daily meal plans with no more than 1,400 calories. She primarily ate salads and burgers and only consumed french fries twice during the 90-day period. Ultimately, she lost 37 pounds. "The problem with a McDonald's-only diet isn't what's on the menu, but the choices made from it," she said afterward. Soso Whaley of Kensington, New Hampshire, made an independent film, *Me and Mickey D*, which chronicled her diet at McDonald's. Over three 30-day periods, she ate only McDonald's food, consuming 2,000 calories per day. She lost 36 pounds, dropping from 175 to 139 pounds.

But such a diet shouldn't be continued long term, and I don't recommend fad-type diets. Human beings benefit from balanced, healthy meals consisting of a variety of nutritious foods. Any type of restrictive diet will probably not provide all of the nutrients, vitamins and minerals that the body needs, nor is it likely to be sustained in the long run. The key is to eat a wide range of nutritious foods in moderation and consume a healthy diet that we can continue for life.

No person who lost weight by eating only fast food is more famous than Jared Fogle, who saw his weight balloon to 425 pounds while attending college. He decided to go on a diet and chose a nearby Subway restaurant to help him do it. He began by skipping breakfast (not something I recommend) and eating only lunch and dinner. He had two sub sandwiches a day, a six-inch turkey sandwich and a large veggie sub. He also ate baked potato chips and diet soda. In one year, Jared dropped to 190 pounds. He has used his success to help others through, among other things, the Jared Foundation, which helps educate kids and their parents and caregivers about the importance of a healthy, balanced diet and exercising regularly. Jared walks the talk. In 2010, he ran and completed the New York City Marathon.

In 2012, Subway received the American Heart Association's Heart-Check Meal certification for some of its meals.

One person who weighed in on those losing weight on a fast food diet was Morgan Spurlock. In *Don't Eat This Book*, he addressed Soso Whaley's McDonald's-only weight-loss program, saying it was hard to believe someone would ever eat an appropriate amount of calories at a fast food restaurant, much less to actually shed weight. "Amazing how that happened, considering she did the two things that no one in America does: *She ate less and exercised.*"

The blanket generalization that *no one* in America eats less and exercises will be news to the millions (although still way too few) who do eat sensibly and exercise regularly. Unfortunately, it's true that many don't engage enough in physical activity. That appears to be changing, albeit slowly. According to the Behavior Risk Factor Surveillance System (the largest telephone survey in the world tracking health risks in the U.S. population), more Americans are exercising, with physical activity rising for both women (+8.6 percent) and men (+3.5 percent) between 2001 and 2007. Is it enough? Absolutely not. We can and must do more. As for eating less, approximately 45 million Americans diet each year, spending almost $2 billion on weight-loss programs. Many of us could do better in these two areas, but there are definitely some who do a great job at both.

Many who aren't successful at weight-loss efforts fail because of the methods they choose. As I've said, and I'm sure you know, diets that are restrictive in calorie or type (for example, low-carb) are typically hard to maintain long term. While there's often an initial weight loss on diets such as these, many people abandon them over time, reverting to their old, bad habits. Many gain back the lost weight *and more*. Sound familiar? That's why it's important to learn how to eat healthfully for life.

In early 2011, Joe the Drive-Thru Runner embarked on a 30-day McDonald's-only diet. Although this is very restrictive, he did it to raise money for the Ronald McDonald House Charities of Chicago and Northwestern Indiana. During this time, he was also training for the L.A. Marathon. His summary of food eaten, total McDonald's visits and miles run: 0 McRibs, 1 Angus Burger, 23 Hamburgers, 24 Chicken Snack Wraps, 14 Fruit & Walnut Salads, 97 Hotcakes, 24 Oatmeals, 23 Cookies, 23 Buckets (soda), 99 Total Visits, 349 Miles Run. Joe came in 28th place at the marathon with a time of 2:36:14, his personal best. He also raised $40,000 for Ronald McDonald House Charities.

A Matter of Choice

Some overweight people have chosen to lay blame on others for their actions: "It's not *my* fault I'm obese…The restaurants did it to me!"

This is perhaps the most disturbing and most dangerous by-product sometimes of the rhetoric of fast food opponents. By laser-focusing their attacks on the sellers of prepared fast food, Spurlock, Schlosser and others may make it easier for some to point a finger at others instead of taking responsibility for our own eating habits. In such cases, I suggest people look within themselves to seek clarity and awareness. Some questions they might ask themselves include:

- Did someone make me eat large quantities of high-fat, high-calorie foods?
- If I am physically able, did someone or something cause me to be more sedentary?
- Do restaurants tell me to overeat or not exercise?
- Do I think that perhaps my food choices, the quantities I choose to eat and my lack of physical activity might be contributors?

Here's another question: what causes us to make unhealthy food choices or not exercise? There are many reasons, and we'll all have different ones and combinations thereof. And some of these are reasonable and even beyond our control. I also know that it can be very hard to motivate ourselves and make changes, no matter how much we want to do it or know that we need it. Sometimes just getting to the point where we acknowledge that we need to make a change can be tough. We're human, after all. And taking personal responsibility for ourselves and our actions isn't always easy and often not very fun. Given that, I have to question if blaming a fast food chain, or any restaurant for that matter, for how we eat is helpful. Just because certain types of food are offered doesn't mean we have to gravitate toward the less healthy choices, or eat too much of even the more-nutritious items. Splurging now and then is fine, but it could pose a definite problem if it happens too often. Fortunately, the power to make the best eating decisions is usually our own. We're driving the car. For most of us, typically our minds, mouths and inactive bodies lead us to a weight problem. But that's not always easy for us to accept.

In 2002, two New Yorkers aged 19 and 14, filed a lawsuit blaming McDonald's Corporation for their high cholesterol, elevated blood pressure, obesity, heart disease and diabetes. They claimed they suffered from these conditions because two McDonald's restaurants in the Bronx didn't "conspicuously disclose the ingredients and effects of its food, including high levels of fat, salt, sugar and cholesterol." This lawsuit was eventually dismissed by Judge Robert Sweet of the U.S. District Court, who ruled that the plaintiffs didn't show that the food at McDonald's was "dangerous in any way other than that which was open and obvious to a reasonable consumer." The judge also didn't find a direct association between the teenagers' health problems and the food at McDonald's. Judge Sweet went on to say, "If a person knows or should know that eating copious orders of supersized McDonald's products is unhealthy and may result in weight gain, it is not the place of the law to protect them from their own excesses."

In 2005, an appeals court gave the lawsuit new life. In the same year, the U.S. House of Representatives passed a bill that banned lawsuits blaming restaurants and food manufacturers for their customers' obesity. The goal of this bill was to rid the clogged civil court system of these types of lawsuits and encourage citizens to take personal responsibility for their actions. As Rep. Chris Cannon of Utah (one of the bill's sponsors) put it, "The bill seeks to block lawsuits by people because they ate too much and got fat." Rep. Lamar Smith of Texas added, "We should not encourage lawsuits that blame others for our own choices and could bankrupt an entire industry."

But that didn't stop another group of overweight citizens from trying their luck with a New York State lawsuit claiming that Burger King, Wendy's, McDonald's and KFC misled them and others by "enticing them with greasy, salty and sugary food." Another plaintive, Caesar Barbar, a diabetic who at one time weighed 275 pounds and had suffered two heart attacks, claimed that fast food had ruined his life. "I always thought it was good for you. I never thought there was anything wrong with it," he said. I definitely feel for him, but remember, like us, he's the quarterback here.

How much fast food Barbar ate wasn't made public, nor was his physical activity level. Remember, moderation and balance are the keys. And it's likely Barbar ate at places other than the fast food restaurants he was suing, including at home.

In response to Barbar's comments, John Doyle, a spokesman for the Center for Consumer Freedom, told ABC News, "He must be aware that fully two-thirds of all foods consumed in America are consumed in people's homes. Is he proposing that we sue America's moms?"

In his book *Fast Food Nation*, Schlosser argues for relieving the individual of responsibility. In his view, we should "resist the seductive argument that people are doing this to themselves, thus justifying inaction." He believes we're the victims of "a finely crafted set of conditions that make it very difficult to eat reasonably and be active."

His points have some merit, but I don't fully buy the argument that we have no power, even in the environments where we live, to eat properly and exercise. True, some of us have a tougher road. Lower-income areas, for example, don't always have a wide variety of healthy food options. Some people might not want to exercise outside in high-crime areas. Also, our lifestyles are so busy that finding time for meals and exercise can be challenging. When these obstacles arise, we need to try to find a way around them or eliminate the problem.

The good news is that the fast food industry, while not to blame for our choices, is helping us make better ones. Sit-down restaurants are joining in on that as well.

McDonald's Corporation recently announced several healthy changes to its menu, marketing and public outreach programs. These include:

- Making the default sides for Happy Meals a half-size order of french fries and a half-size order of apple slices.

This reduced Happy Meal calories by approximately 20 percent. Patrons have the opportunity to have only a full-size order of either fries or apple slices as a side. Unfortunately, only about 11 percent of customers request apple slices with the Happy Meals.

- Including nutrition and/or "active lifestyle" information on Happy Meal packaging and in television, magazine and digital advertising.
- Providing nutrition awareness programs in communities.
- Reducing calories, added sugars and saturated fat in menu items by 2020.
- Reducing sodium content of its national menu items an average of 15 percent by the year 2015.

McDonald's has also teamed with Weight Watchers in 150 restaurants in New Zealand. Some menu items are assigned 6.5 points for Kiwi diners following the Weight Watchers point program. In Australia, more than 745 McDonald's restaurants joined with the National Heart Foundation's Tick program. Nine meals were chosen for the foundation's "tick of approval." Fifteen percent of customers bought these healthier menu options, the foundation found.

McDonald's isn't alone in offering healthy initiatives. In 2011, the National Restaurant Association kicked off its Kids LiveWell program in the United States. More than 15,000 restaurants from 19 brands participate—fast food restaurants and conventional sit-down restaurants alike—including Outback Steakhouse, Chili's Grill & Bar, Corner Bakery Café, El Pollo Loco, Burger King, Carrabba's Italian Grill, T-Bones Great American Eatery, zpizza, Au Bon Pain, Cracker Barrel, Friendly's, Chevys Fresh Mex, Bonefish Grill, IHOP, Denny's, Silver Diner and Sizzler. The program's criteria for healthier menu options include:

- Offering a minimum of one individual food item of 200 calories or less, with a limit on sugar, sodium and fat, plus a serving of vegetables, fruit, lean protein or low-fat dairy and whole grains.
- Providing a kids meal that includes an entrée, side and a drink, two servings of vegetables, fruit, whole grains, lean protein and/or dairy containing 600 calories or less. As with the individual food item, limits would be in place on fat, sugar and sodium content.
- Including nutrition information on the healthy menu offerings.

One new trend is that of some fast food restaurants selling alcohol. Recently, several Sonic restaurants in South Florida announced that they'd be joining some of Starbuck's Seattle stores in selling wine and beer. And Burger King sells beer at "Whopper Bars" in Kansas City, Las Vegas and Miami. Remember, moderation is the key and drive safely!

In 2012, the Kids LiveWell program received the American Society of Association Executive Gold Circle Award. This award recognizes innovation and excellence in communications.

While McDonald's and other fast food establishments have responded to the demand for healthier food choices, it's true they still offer less-nutritious menu selections. But of course, so do all types of restaurants, from casual dining to fine dining. And make no mistake about it: Eating excessive quantities of fat- and cholesterol-laden calories is bad for you, no matter where you get them. We can also make unhealthy choices when eating at home, sitting down to a business luncheon, at a party, or just about any place that we eat. If we make an effort to eat sensibly most of the time, an occasional cheeseburger and french fries is still okay. It's about balance and moderation.

Todd G. Buchholz, author of *Burger, Fries and Lawyers: The Beef Behind Obesity Laws*, sets up a scenario that questions the obesity blame game. Here's his interesting perspective:

> A scene: The overweight baseball fan jumps to his feet in the bleachers of Wrigley Field, screaming for the Chicago Cubs to hold onto their 3-2 lead in the bottom of the ninth inning. He squeezes a Cubs pennant in his left hand while shoving a mustard-smeared hot dog in his mouth with the right. The Dodgers have a runner on first, who is sneaking a big lead off the base. The Cubs' pitcher has thrown three balls and two strikes to the batter, a notorious power hitter. The obese fan holds his breath while the pitcher winds up and fires a blazing fastball. "Crack!" The ball flies over the fan's head into the bleachers for a game-winning home run. The fan slumps to his bleacher seat and has a heart attack.
>
> Whom should the fan sue? (a) The Cubs for breaking his heart? (b) The hot dog company for making a fatty food? (c) The hot dog vendor for selling him a fatty food? (d) All of the above.

I ask, how about taking responsibility for himself and his actions? The correct answer is he should sue himself.

FOUR

Get off the Couch!

"More than 80 percent of adults do not meet the guidelines for both aerobic and muscle-strengthening activities. Similarly, more than 80 percent of adolescents do not do enough aerobic physical activity to meet the guidelines for youth."

—**U.S. Department of Health and Human Services**
Physical Activity Guidelines for Americans

Who remembers the Special K commercial back in the day that told us if we could pinch an inch of our abdomen, we had some work to do? Who can pinch way more than that? A lot of us. Who's looked in the mirror and asked, "Who's this person staring back at me? It can't actually be me." I suspect more than a few of us have been there.

How about seeing important health indicators such as cholesterol, blood sugar and blood pressure rise beyond the normal range? Working in a hospital, I know that this is more than a few of us unfortunately. As already mentioned, a lot of us have seen our weights rise beyond what they should be. And those of us whose body weights are in a healthy range aren't always as fit and healthy as we could be. People of all shapes and sizes can get sick and experience lifestyle-related disease.

So what's the problem? Besides watching what we eat, what can we do? Let me ask you this, who among us at this exact moment can easily go out and walk a brisk three miles…or even one mile? Is it dawning on you where I'm going next?

You got it—food isn't the only component in weight gain. So is exercise, or the lack thereof. People who are physically able but don't exercise can potentially open themselves up to many health risks, including obesity and chronic disease. People who don't exercise are almost twice as likely to develop heart disease compared to those who work out regularly. Although the numbers are improving, only around 22 percent of adults in the United States vigorously exercise at least 20 minutes or more, three or more times per week. This percentage lowers to only about 15 percent of those who exercise at least 30 minutes five days or more per week. Not good. But worse is the approximately 40 percent of adult Americans who don't engage in any vigorous physical activity at all. We are a busy, yet sedentary society. The outcome is too many calories in and too few calories out. As a result, many of us are overweight or obese.

Minimally, adults should exercise for at least 30 minutes, five days per week. This helps us to manage chronic disease, but typically isn't enough to result in weight loss. To melt away pounds, 60 to 90 minutes of physical activity most days of the week is recommended. Children and adolescents benefit from exercise and should aim for at least 60 minutes of physical activity daily.

Walk a Mile in Those Shoes

Americans' love of inactivity now begins early in life. Only about half of those aged 12 to 21 exercise vigorously on a regular basis. And only around 25 percent engage in even light to moderate physical activity (for example, bicycling, walking) almost daily. This means a large segment of this population isn't moving. It's never too late to embark on an exercise program. Every day, I encounter many adults of all ages, from 25 to 85 plus, who are just beginning a workout regimen. I also see children and adolescents starting sporting activities and the like. This will do many good things for them. Starting at any age is great, but introducing regular physical activity at a young age is especially positive.

Many of us have a difficult time starting and/or maintaining a physical activity program. Some of us don't have a lot of time. Others have physical issues that limit the type of exercise they can engage in. And, there are some of us who just don't like to sweat or feel uncomfortable among more fit bodies at a gym. These are real issues, but they're not insurmountable.

- If you have limited time, try exercising in ten-minute intervals several times a day.
- It's difficult for many of us to do, but try getting up a little earlier to get some activity into your day.

- If you feel uncomfortable in a gym environment, exercise at home. DVDs/videos, Wii and similar computer games, exercise equipment, or a walk around the neighborhood are all good things to try.
- If you have limited mobility, try things like chair exercising, yoga, swimming, or any other type of exercise that you can comfortably do.
- If you don't like to sweat, at least exercise in a time frame that allows you to shower soon after finishing your workout.
- Find an exercise buddy to help motivate you.
- Team sports are always a great option.

The point is to just start doing something. I recently spoke with a man who decided he would start playing Ping-Pong as his form of exercise. He would play up to several hours per day. What a great idea. Did he burn calories? You bet he did, about 300 every hour he played. And you know he had fun doing it.

If I don't exercise, not only do I not feel as good, my waistline suffers. So, I work to incorporate exercise into my life on a regular basis. It isn't always easy, but I try my best. Even so, it took me a bit of time to find my "rhythm" in the physical activity arena. I've joined a gym many times, only to never go. I finally realized I don't want to get into a car and drive to go exercise. It's just too hard for me. Conversely, my husband drives to the gym at least three days a week and has done so for years. It works for him. We're all different and will approach our workouts accordingly. What was the solution to my not-wanting-to-exercise-outside-of-the-home dilemma? I bought a treadmill and it's worked out great for me.

It's important that we do what we like when exercising and choose times that are convenient for us. It helps us stick with it. I also like to add in a motivator. I wear the digital pedometer called the Fitbit. I adore it. Besides telling me how many steps/miles I've walked, how many stairs I've climbed, and how many calories I've burned, it gives me messages that make me laugh. The other day I picked it up and the readout said, "Hug me. Go Lisa!" And go I did. One day I walked more than 15,000 steps and it emailed me a congratulatory note.

I love any type of pedometer, from the more basic to my higher-tech. They tend to spur us on. Aim for 10,000 steps per day, or five miles. If it takes time to get there, no problem. Just work up to it.

Because most of my physical activity revolves around walking, I recently decided to mix things up. I bought the cutest pink bicycle and tricked it out with a floral basket, streamers and paisley helmet. The first time I got on it and started riding around my neighborhood I felt like I was sty-lin'! This euphoria lasted for the eight minutes that my legs did, until they didn't want to peddle anymore. Having not ridden a bike for about 30 years, eight minutes was all I could do. I didn't let that deter me. It became my starting point and over weeks and months I built up my biking time to a respectable one.

Whatever we can do to be physically active is so important, because as you can see below, there's no denying it's good for us.

With all these proven benefits of regular exercise, it amazes me that more of us aren't physically active. Just take a look at this list:
1. Weight loss
2. Improve flexibility
3. Increase muscle mass
4. Improve endurance
5. Increase energy
6. Increase bone density
7. Reduce blood sugar
8. Improve sleep
9. Reduce stress
10. Increase good HDL and decrease LDL

There are so many ways children and adolescents today can be entertained without having to move their limbs. At the risk of dating myself, computers, console games and even VCRs (yes, VCRs) didn't exist when I was a kid. Aside from wondering what Buffy and Jody or the Beaver were going to get themselves into on the tube, there wasn't much of anything else that kept a kid sedentary. We walked and ran, rode bikes and played basketball, baseball, softball and tetherball on a regular basis. Unlike today, when many schools have cut back on their physical education programs, P.E. classes and recess were the norm in years past. In 2006, less than 50 percent of school kids were exposed to physical education classes on a daily basis. And we wonder why our children are gaining unnecessary weight.

Today's culture is different. The average child in America between 8 and 18 spends approximately 44.5 hours a week watching television or sitting at their computers. These kids watch about 1,680 minutes of television a week. The only thing that consumes more of their time is sleeping.

> Of polled 4-to-6-year-olds, 54 percent said if they had to choose, they'd rather watch TV than spend time with their fathers.

There have been more than 4,000 studies focused on the effects of television on children, and more than a few of these have examined the relationship between TV viewership levels and childhood obesity. One study found that children who watched in excess of three hours of television each day had a 50 percent greater likelihood of being obese than those children watching less than two hours. The study noted that more than 60 percent of overweight cases can be linked to excess TV viewing.

- Other studies have had similar findings as follows:

- Data from a national survey between 1998 and 2004 reported that 26 percent of kids watching at least four or more hours of TV a day had much greater body fat than those who watched less television.

- A study of children aged 1 to 4 indicated that each hour of daily television viewing was associated with a *6 percent increase* in obesity risk. If the kid had a television in his or her own room, the odds that he/she would be overweight dramatically *increased by 31 percent* for every hour of TV watching.

To make matters worse, children today don't even have to walk to go places. They can now roll. A big pet peeve of mine is the tennis shoes with wheels, or Heelys. These "shoes" reduce the need for kids to use their legs to get from point A to point B; now they can simply glide along. They aren't roller skates or bicycles, yet they're not just athletic shoes. Perhaps

---

Physical Activity Guidelines for Americans

The following guidelines are from the U.S. Department of Health and Human Services:

Children and Adolescents: This group should engage in at least one hour (60 minutes) of exercise every day, mostly through moderate to vigorous aerobic activity. Vigorous intensity activity should be engaged in at least three times per week, as should muscle/bone strengthening activity.

Adults: At a minimum, adults should engage in at least 2 hours and 30 minutes of moderate intensity aerobic exercise per week (or 1 hour and 15 minutes of vigorous intensity aerobic activity). Aerobic activity should be in increments of at least ten minute sessions.

Muscle strengthening exercises should be done at least two days per week.

there's a slight benefit for balancing and stretching, but who on earth thought this was a good idea? Heelys were responsible for about 1,600 emergency room visits in 2006 and many venues such as schools, libraries, shopping centers and amusement parks have banned them. And adults, we're not off the hook either. All I need to say is "Segway," the world's "first self-balancing human transporter." We, too, don't have to walk. In fact, if both adults and children continue on this course, we'll be exactly like the comically obese humans depicted in the Pixar movie *WALL-E*, who floated through their daily lives on moving recliners and were so out of shape that they could barely stand on their own.

The childhood obesity statistics (as well as adult ones) are alarming and the link to inactivity can't be denied. Now here's the $64,000 question: Do fast food restaurants have anything at all to do with the amount of time that children (and let's be honest, us adults) sit in front of televisions, computers, iPads, PlayStations or other media? We all know that they don't. Could personal responsibility, schools and paternal oversight perhaps come in to play here? We all know that they do.

If anything, the fast food industry supports athletics and physical activities. Many restaurants have "play places" where children can be physically active in a safe and clean environment. Major fast food chains also associate and advertise with professional athletes, sporting teams and arenas. McDonald's is even a major sponsor of the Olympics.

For the 2012 London Olympic Games, McDonald's opened a two-story, 3,000- square-meter restaurant, its largest freestanding unit in the world, right in Olympic Park. As part of its Champions of Play program, a global initiative to help promote "a balanced approach to nutrition and activity for children," McDonald's brought 200 kids from all around the globe to London. They were able to participate in a variety of activities, including spending time with the athletes.

Opponents might say fast food restaurants shouldn't be placed in the same sentence, room, or galaxy as athletic pursuits. It's advertising to generate sales, for sure, but perhaps there's a larger effect. For a child to see the golden arches or Ronald McDonald associated with an athlete, sport, or particular gaming event, certainly gives the

As part of its 2012 Olympics promotions, McDonald's announced it "Favorites Under 400" menu in the United States. Approximatçely 80% of its items are less than 400 calories. But, french fries are part of this menu, so again make healthier choices most of the time.

sponsoring corporation a "halo effect." But it can also work the other way. Whether intentionally or not, these companies are sending the message that sports are good and worthwhile. However, they should showcase healthier menu choices when using athletes to promote their food. I was disappointed when McDonald's showed athletes eating their new Southern Style Fried Chicken Sandwiches during the 2008 Olympic Games. Frying, after all, isn't a healthy form of food preparation.

Nike sums it up best with its slogan, "Just Do It." Getting started can be tough, but once we begin, it can be become a habit and a good one at that!

FIVE

Is It a Ban...or a Band-Aid?

"There is a correlation between obesity and lower income, but it cannot be solely attributed to restaurant choice...Obesity among the poor is more due to the relatively cheap price of junk food items found in supermarkets, convenience stores and mom-and-pop markets in impoverished neighborhoods."

—J. Paul Leigh, professor of public health sciences at UC Davis

In the past several years, some cities in California have taken steps to stem the tide of the obesity epidemic. That's great. Helping people understand the mechanics of a healthy lifestyle and how to make better choices would benefit all. But unfortunately, education isn't the path these cities took. Instead, they called out "the ban." The targets were both fast food locations and free kids' toys with meals.

To Dine or Not to Dine

New fast food restaurants have been banned from lower-income South Los Angeles. In 2011, approximately 30 percent of the 750,000 residents in the affected area were obese. This was about double the obesity rate found in higher-income areas of Los Angeles. At the time, there were close to 1,000 fast food restaurants in the approximate 30-square-mile area that came under the regulation. Proponents of the regulation wanted more sit-down restaurants and grocery stores loaded with fresh produce and healthy foods. But sit-down restaurants have menu offerings that are loaded with calories, fat and sodium. Mom-and-pop eating establishments can be perpetrators of high-calorie concoctions and grocery stores also sell many unhealthy items. And while the ban has been in effect since 2008, as of early 2011 only one new grocery store had opened in the affected area.

Proponents of the fast food ban say fast food is bad for you, just like drinking or smoking. It can be, but it doesn't have to be. A local activist group, Community Coalition, likens this ban to tightening controls on liquor stores, seedy motels and other "nuisance businesses." I don't agree, nor do I think such a ban will solve the obesity epidemic.

In 2009, a RAND Corporation research group study found that the fast food ban wasn't likely to change the obesity rates or associated lifestyle diseases such as diabetes in the regulated area. It suggested that unhealthy snacks found at convenience stores and gas stations should receive more focus. As study co-author and RAND senior economist Roland Sturm put it, "People get a lot more of their discretionary and unnecessary food from there than from a fast-food restaurant...People talk about this area being a food desert, but it is more like a swamp— you are literally drowning in food, but none of it is really a good option."

According to the U.S. Agriculture Research Service, approximately 90 percent of Americans snack between meals, double the intake from 30 years ago. And we're making it easier to get snacks. The new trend is drive-thru windows at convenience stores.

When the ordinance first went in to effect, its sponsor, Los Angeles Councilwoman Jan Perry, said, "This ordinance is in no way attempting to tell people what to eat but rather responding to the need to attract sit-down restaurants, full service grocery stores and healthy food alternatives. Ultimately, this ordinance is about providing choices—something that is currently lacking in our community."

Councilwoman Perry's plan may not work as intended. A 15-year study of thousands of people found that improved availability to grocery stores didn't lead to healthier diets. In fact, the study group participants didn't consume any more vegetables and fruits when they had convenient access to supermarkets.

Interestingly, a recent study conducted by two health economics specialists from UC-Davis Center for Healthcare Policy and Research found that visits to fast food restaurants actually became more frequent as household incomes increased. This was true up to a household income of $60,000. Above that, visits to fast food restaurants decreased.

FAST FOOD VINDICATION

When I worked for McDonald's Corporation, I leased a free-standing location in the parking lot of a shopping center. Part of the building would be a coffee shop and McDonald's would occupy the other half. The location was on a very busy street in an area densely populated with residents and businesses. On one side of the boulevard was a low-income area. On the other side there were high-end neighborhoods. It couldn't have been more polarized. A public hearing was required to get all the permits needed and both groups came out. The high-income residents were not in support of the project for the most part. They arrived in Mercedes, Jaguars and BMWs. The lower-income residents came together in the local church bus. Many of them didn't have their own transportation. This group was in support of the project.

The wealthy group was against McDonald's going into the center for reasons that had nothing to do with food or nutrition. The lower-income group spoke only about the food. They talked about McDonald's being an affordable restaurant where they could feed their families. Close walking proximity and a safe play area also made the list. The site was located near all types of restaurants and an ample supply of grocery and specialty food stores. Even with all that choice, the lower-income group took time out of their day to travel downtown to a public hearing to help fight for another fast food restaurant to come into their neighborhood.

South Los Angeles may also find that stopping fast food establishments from building new locations doesn't achieve the intended result. In a 2011 article for the *New York Times*, Jennifer Medina wrote that a Carl's Jr. located in South Los Angeles was packed the afternoon that she was there. One mother there with her two children eating fried Chicken Stars told Medina, "This is a fun thing for them and easy for me, so how can I not come at least once a week or something like that? When you're out, you are just going to look for the first decent thing around. If there are fewer of them, fine by me, but we're still going to go to the ones we've got now."

It's fine that this mother and her children go to any fast food restaurant. Or anyone for that matter. People will always go to them, even if they're restricted or limited by local ordinances. What concerns me is what people are ordering most of the time at *any* type of restaurant. I'm not a fan of fried Chicken Stars; I'm a grilled chicken girl all the way. For me, the takeaway is education about making healthier choices. This would serve us far better than moratoriums like the one South Los Angeles imposed.

At the time of the fast food ban, I asked Jim Carras, vice president of Real Estate for McDonald's US, if the corporation had any concerns. He said no. He also didn't believe limiting fast food growth would affect the so-called "food deserts." In fact, he said the presence of McDonald's and other high-volume restaurants on shared properties would actually be a draw for supermarkets that might otherwise be hesitant to locate in lower-income areas.

It doesn't appear overall the ban had a significant effect on larger corporations. While not growing locations in the banned area, McDonald's is still adding locations in the U.S., including Los Angeles. And in 2011, the corporation reported a 4.8 percent increase in same store sales, its best return since 2006.

The other fast food chains are growing as well. David Novak, CEO of Yum Brands (Taco Bell, KFC and Pizza Hut) said that in 2012 the company hoped to see something like a 5 percent growth rate in the United States in 2012. He sees Yum Brands as a global company, with over 70 percent of its 2011 profits coming from restaurants located outside of the United States.

South Los Angeles isn't the only area in Southern California that has tried to stop the fast food giants in their tracks. In early 2012, Loma Linda, which has the nation's largest congregation of Seventh-Day Adventists, saw many of its citizens rise up in an attempt to stop a recently approved McDonald's, citing religious beliefs as the reason. This was despite the fact that other fast food outlets like Carl's Jr., Del Taco and KFC currently have locations in Loma Linda.

Seventh-Day Adventists believe in a healthy lifestyle and many are vegetarians. Among other things, they typically don't smoke or drink alcohol or caffeinated beverages, focusing on eating nuts, grains, fruits, and vegetables. They also believe in an active lifestyle. And it seems to pay off. Researchers at Loma Linda University found that the lifespan of Seventh-Day Adventists is longer than the general population by almost five years for females and over seven years for males. And it's easy to see why: Eating nutritious foods, exercising, and avoiding unhealthy activities are great ingredients for longevity.

But while some of the Loma Linda residents may believe McDonald's symbolizes unhealthiness, not all of them think that banning a particular restaurant is the right thing to do. "I don't think we should be getting into the business of legislating vegetarianism," said Rhodes Rigsby, mayor of Loma Linda and assistant dean of the Loma Linda University School of Medicine. And 95-year-old Dr. Ellsworth Wareham, a long-time vegan (eating no animal products) who retired from his career as a heart surgeon at age 93, showed a common-sense approach when he said, "I don't subscribe to the menu that these dear people put out, but let's face it, the average eating place serves food that is, let us say, a little bit of a higher quality, but the end result is the same—it's unhealthy… They can put it right next to the church as far as I am concerned." Again, it's about personal responsibility and making better choices.

People for the Ethical Treatment of Animals (PETA) appears to share in the sentiment that a meatless world is the goal. I asked Eric Deardorff, PETA Action Team coordinator, why they target fast food restaurants, particularly McDonald's, for their various campaigns, to the seeming exclusion of other restaurants that sell animal products. He explained that McDonald's is one of their "main campaign targets" because of its size and amount of chicken sales. PETA also "would like for all restaurants to serve plant-based foods exclusively because of the effects of meat, dairy and eggs on animals, human health, and the environment. However, we know that won't happen overnight and so we push for pragmatic changes while pursuing our goal." It's important for all restaurants to do what they can to improve animal welfare, but being a vegetarian is a very specific choice and shouldn't be mandated for any.

Vegetarianism can be a very healthy way of eating. There are many potential benefits of eschewing animal protein for plant proteins, such as lower cholesterol levels, lower blood pressure, reduced insulin needs for insulin-dependent individuals, lower incidence of some cancers, lower risk of osteoporosis and a lower tendency of getting kidney stonesor gallstones, among others. But being a vegetarian isn't for everyone. In fact, it's not for a lot of people.

In many of the classes that I teach, I ask if anyone is vegetarian. It's rare that anyone says they are. If I told the thousands of people who have said they eat animal products that they couldn't have them, I would receive a great deal of push back. So many of us enjoy them and won't give them up. Certainly there are high-fat meat choices and methods of food preparation. But there are also healthy animal product choices. Fish, skinless white meat poultry, egg whites, low-fat/non-fat milk—when prepared in a healthy manner and in appropriate portion size—are fine for most. Denial doesn't work well for a lot of us, including me. Making healthier choices within all the food groups that we eat is easier to manage.

The reasons for attacks on fast food restaurants are indeed varied. In August 1999, French activist Jose Bové and several others literally took apart a McDonald's that was under construction in the city of Millau. Their purpose was to protest U.S. tariffs on French cheese. In a 2001 interview, Bové discussed his being made somewhat of a hometown hero for this: "The protest went along and everybody, including the kids, helped dismantle the interior of the building: partitions, some doors, electrical outlets, and sheet metal on the roof...Everything was put into two tractor wagons...Both wagons were full, one of them a grain dumpster. Some of the kids leaving the site climbed into the dumpster with pieces of wood in their hands to pretend to play drums, and we all took off in a

cont. on page 64

cont. from page 63

parade toward police headquarters in Millau. There was clapping as we rode through the city: people thought it was funny and fun. We unloaded the wagons in front of the police station…To show that we didn't think that it was any big deal to dismantle a fast food place, I went on vacation right after the event."

I don't know about you, but I think that vandalism and theft *are* a big deal, and, of course, wrong and illegal. Protests can be important and effective, but the destruction of property isn't the way to go.

Many people enjoy eating at fast food restaurants. In the case of college football linebacker Cassanova McKinzy, one of his stated reasons for choosing Auburn over Clemson had to do with a certain fast food restaurant. In explaining his choice of not attending Clemson, McKinzy said it was "kind of the environment and plus they had no Chick-fil-A on campus." (It turns out, though, that Clemson does indeed have a Chick-fil-A.)

Often, stores sell less-healthy items without anyone seemingly having a problem with it. In Beverly Hills, California, there's a store called Sprinkles that sells cupcakes. The demand for them is so great that owner Candace Nelson (also a judge on the Food Network show *Cupcake Wars*) installed a vending machine, or "Cupcake ATM" as Sprinkles calls it, for people to more readily get this dessert. It's *24-hour*, no less, and dispenses about 1,000 cupcakes a day. Nine other cities, including Chicago and New York, are slated to get their own ATMs of the cupcake variety. On the day their New York availability was announced, there didn't appear to be any alarm bells raised, only happy, excited comments. "You can never have too much access to your cupcakes," said a visitor at the New York Sprinkles. Is a cupcake every now and then okay? Sure. But I wonder, if a fast food restaurant had opened up a vending machine selling their cookies or pies, would the response would have been as benevolent?

We may soon know the answer to this question. While not exactly fast food, pizza has entered the world of vending machines. Already operating in Europe and soon to come to the U.S., the machines spit out a quick-cooked, 10.5-inch pepperoni, ham, bacon or margherita pizza with 676 calories and 22.6 g of fat.

Brother, Can You Spare a Dime?

In late 2010, San Francisco banned free toys with children's meals at fast food restaurants that didn't meet nutritional criteria in the city's Healthy Food Incentives Ordinance. This came after nearby Santa Clara County's ban. San Francisco's ordinance prohibits free toys with children's meals if the food and beverage provided combined have more than 600 calories and more than 35 percent of total calories from fat. Restaurants are also required to provide fruits and vegetables with all kids' meals that come with toys.

In 2011, New York City Councilman Leroy Comrie proposed a similar ban on fast food toys with meals. There was some backlash. Alison Gartner, a mother of two, said, "I feel that it is the parent's decision of whether they want to give a child a Happy Meal or not and it really shouldn't involve a councilman." McDonald's Regional Vice President Mason Smoot responded, "We provide options for our customers and trust them to make the decisions that are right for their families. Politicians should too." Smoot added, "On average, kids eat at McDonald's about three times a month; that means about 87 other meals are eaten at home, school or elsewhere. That adds up to a discussion larger than toys."

In response to San Francisco's fast food toy ban, *SF Weekly* reported that "the school lunches our children eat aren't healthy enough to qualify." Although strides have been made in the nutritional value of school meals, french fries are still on the menu and pizza still counts as a vegetable. An adult staffer of the Rethink program echoed that sentiment in the HBO documentary series, *The Weight of the Nation*: "We treat schools and young people as the garbage disposals of America."

In addition, "pink slime"—a concoction of cow intestines, connective tissue and cartilage not found in typical cuts of beef, and which have been found to be more vulnerable to E. coli and salmonella—is still being served in schools, although the USDA recently announced that they will give schools the choice of an alternative ground beef option. While some schools will still serve pink slime, Burger King, Taco Bell and McDonald's decided to stop using it.

Interestingly, while many school districts no longer serve chocolate milk, something that I applaud, the dairy industry didn't pack it up. They now market it to adult athletes with basketball pro Carmelo Anthony and Olympic swimming medalist Dara Torres as spokespersons. I would consider chocolate milk a treat, not something anybody should drink on a regular basis. Remember, moderation is key. Low-fat and non-fat milk are the healthier choices.

So, were the bans effective? As far as Santa Clara County's goes, sort of. A January 2012 article in the *American Journal of Preventative Medicine* found that while the affected restaurants did make some changes with regard to promoting healthy meals and nutrition, they didn't change menu items or add new ones. They just promoted already existing healthier menu options.

In San Francisco, McDonald's found a way to stay within the ordinance's parameters by charging a dime for a toy when a Happy Meal is purchased. The proceeds go to Ronald McDonald House, which helps families with sick children.

So the ordinances didn't seem to serve their intended purpose. But if they had, would it have been the answer? Probably not. As one skeptic, Albert Einstein College of Medicine associate professor of pediatrics Keith Ayoob, put it, "It's misguided to think that this is going to combat childhood obesity. We should be focusing on school lunches, where there are a lot more calories and fat than Happy Meals, and what kids are eating at home." In Ayoob's view, the politicians behind such bans instead "...should be doing something like mandating physical education for all grades in the school system." I say definitely do that and make sure there's health education for both the students and the parents. And the food at sit-down restaurants should also be examined.

One ban I don't take issue with is the trans fat ban instituted by cities such as New York and Baltimore. Trans fat, or hydrogenated fat, is made when polyunsaturated fat is processed and becomes solid at room temperature. This makes it more saturated, which can raise the level of cholesterol in the blood. Trans fat is is found in products such as lard; margarine; vegetable shortening; baked goods such as cookies, chips and crackers; and other processed foods. It's a hidden ingredient many consumers don't know is in the product. And it's not

cont. on page 68

cont. from page 67

good for us. Trans fat can increase LDL (bad cholesterol) levels and decrease HDL (good cholesterol) levels. Some cities are now also going after the high sodium content of foods. I support this. High sodium intake can be harmful. Removing unhealthy ingredients and replacing them with healthier ones isn't a bad trend.

Recently, New York City Mayor Michael Bloomberg announced a proposal to ban sales of sugary drinks larger than 16 ounces. The targeted beverages are those sweetened with sugar or another type of caloric sweetener containing more than 25 calories per eight fluid ounces. This ban would exclude diet soda and drinks that are at least half milk or milk substitute-based. Reactions have been mixed. "I like Mayor Bloomberg, but are you kidding me?" said U.S. House of Representatives Speaker John Boehner. "Come on, don't we have bigger issues to deal with than the size of soft drinks somebody buys?"

No one hit that nail more squarely on the head than late-night television host Jon Stewart, who demonstrated the potential ineffectiveness of limiting the size of drinks while not taking into account the often large calorie counts of a variety of menu items at various New York eateries.

In Stewart's piece, he sipped from a large-sized Slurpee and lamented how Bloomberg's proposal would affect it. Good news for Stewart and other Slurpee fans: Not only does the ban not apply to convenience stores (only to establishments that require a health inspection report, such as restaurants, movie theaters, food carts and sports venues), but in June 2012, 7-Eleven started selling Slurpee Lite, lowering calories through the use of Splenda. The first flavor sold nationwide was Sugar-Free Mango with 20 calories in an eight-ounce serving.

One of the calorie-laden dishes showcased in Jon Stewart's bit was a sandwich from a famous New York deli that was so thick with meat probably no human jaw could open wide enough to take a bite from it as served. You've probably seen a sandwich like this in your day. And the phenomenon of very large sandwiches isn't limited to the United States. In Japan, Burger King offered a promotion in which customers could add 15 strips of bacon to any sandwich for 100 yen, or $1.20 U.S. The promotion could be applied 70 times per sandwich, and at least one person took advantage by ordering 1,050 bacon slices for his burger. The resulting $80 Whopper had a reported 74,170 calories. So in this case, the size of the soda wasn't the biggest issue.

In June 2012, Cambridge, Massachusetts, Mayor Henrietta Davis unveiled a policy resolution that would ban sugar-laden beverages and sodas. This would be a complete ban, not reducing serving sizes like New York aims to do. This isn't sitting well with many residents. One pondered: "So zero soda, but I could order an entire pizza? It's pathetic."

Coca-Cola is fighting Mayor Bloomberg's plan to limit soda sizes. Katie Bayne, the soft-drink giant's president of sparkling beverages said sugar intake from beverages actually *declined* from 1999 to 2010, at a time that obesity was rising. "Sugars from soda consumption fell 39% even as the percentage of obese kids jumped 13% and obese adults climbed 7%."

While this may be the case, drinks shouldn't account for a lot of calories in the diet. With the exception of milk, try to aim for 30 calories or less per beverage. Zero (for example, water) is better.

A Picture Is Worth a Thousand Words

Another recent push has been to ban fast food commercials on TV. The 65,000-member strong American Academy of Pediatrics (AAP) is looking to do just that. Dr. Victor Strasburger, author of the new AAP policy, explained: "It's time for the food industry to clean up its act and not advertise junk food to young children. Just by banning ads for fast food, one study says we could decrease obesity and overweight by 17 percent."

An interagency government group is working on voluntary guidelines for self-regulation by food companies and restaurants "to improve the nutritional profile of foods most heavily marketed to children." Already, companies such as General Mills, Kraft Foods Global, PepsiCo, McDonald's and Kellogg's are working with the Better Business Bureau to reduce their marketing to kids.

One food that's often marketed to children (and adults alike) is breakfast cereal. Some of these cereals contain a lot of sugar. A recent survey by the Environmental Working Group found that one cup of Apple Jacks or Cap'n Crunch Cereal contains more sugar than three Chips Ahoy cookies. The worst offender in the study was Kellogg's Honey Smacks, which has more sugar in one cup (5 teaspoons) than a Hostess Twinkie. Should we avoid cereals? Of course not. They can be a good source of fiber and vitamins and minerals. Better cereals cited in the study, with less than a quarter teaspoon of sugar, included: Post Shredded Wheat, Cheerios (original), and unfrosted bite-sized Kellogg's Mini-Wheats. If you check the labels on the boxes in the cereal aisle, you'll find many more low-sugar choices.

In mid-2012, the Walt Disney Company announced that by 2015 all advertising on Disney Channel, Disney Junior, Disney XD, Radio Disney and Disney.com, as well as Saturday morning children-oriented programs on ABC-owned stations, would follow Disney's guidelines for nutrition with regard to limiting calories, saturated fat, sugar and sodium.

Some advertisements about fast food are intended to scare us away. In 2010, the Physicians Committee for Responsible Medicine designed an ad that became known as the "McDonald's Death Ad" or the "Consequences clip." In a morgue, we see a lady crying over a man's dead body, which is holding a sandwich from McDonald's. There were some strong opinions about the ad, including from McDonald's. "This commercial is outrageous, misleading and unfair to all consumers," said Bridget Coffing, vice president of global communications for the company. "McDonald's trusts our customers to put such outlandish propaganda in perspective, and to make food and lifestyle choices that are right for them."

PETA is also known for its graphic ads and campaigns. In a pedestrian retail area known as Third Street Promenade in Santa Monica, California, I was able to see first-hand the very disturbed parents and children who were subjected to a video of animals in slaughterhouses produced by the group. I was there to view the McDonald's location scheduled to open the next day and PETA was there to protest the event. The video was quite graphic and there were many unhappy families—and it wasn't McDonald's they were angry at. It was PETA.

PETA has also angered parents in other areas. Albany, New York is one such place. Parents took exception to PETA's "McCruelty Campaign," saying that they didn't like their children seeing pictures of chickens being slaughtered. Who can blame them.

FAST FOOD VINDICATION

I'm a firm believer in humane treatment of animals. This is a topic worthy of scrutiny. But filters are important, particularly when children are involved. In this case, PETA's demonstration may not have elicited the response it was aiming for.

We've seen that the fast food industry has become a scapegoat in a number of areas, based largely on a lack of knowledge about the companies, their history and actual business practices. It's worthwhile, then, to take a closer look at these institutions and the unique place they have come to occupy in society.

Six

The Growth of an Industry

"Only in America, would a guy like me, from humble beginnings and without a high school diploma become successful. America gave me a chance to live the life I want and work to make my dreams come true. We should never take our freedoms for granted, and we should seize every opportunity presented to us."

—Dave Thomas, founder of Wendy's

A common refrain of the fast food industry's critics is that the sheer size of the companies is something to be feared. They have become too powerful, and their influence has become too pervasive in society. In his books *Fast Food Nation* and *Chew on This* (co-authored by Charles Wilson), Eric Schlosser speaks often on this point. In *Fast Food Nation*, he provides a list of facts presented in a negative light. However, with a different viewpoint, many can just as easily be seen as positives:

- Approximately one out of eight people in the U.S. work force has been employed by McDonald's at some time in their lives.
- In 2001, McDonald's was responsible for 90 percent of the new jobs in America.
- McDonald's hires more people (approximately 1 million each year) than any other company in America.
- McDonald's buys more chicken, beef, pork, apples and potatoes than any other U.S. company.
- In 2001, McDonald's restaurants had more children's play areas than any other private entity in America.
- McDonald's ranks as one of America's largest toy distributors.

Play areas? Toys? Jobs? How dare they! Schlosser depicts the fast food industry as an insidious force that works its many tentacles into the very fabric of society. But is it so wrong, especially during troubled economic times, to employ more people than any other U.S. company? Or to purchase large quantities of wholesale food products, to say nothing of fixtures, refrigeration equipment and packaging materials?

In April 2011, McDonald's announced that it would hire 50,000 new employees in one day. Providing employment to this number of people amounted to a 7 percent increase in the company's total workforce—an average of about four new employees at each restaurant. The starting pay was about $8 per hour, and managers could earn $50,000 a year. As reported by ABC News, the impact of this hiring blitz could result in those new workers pumping over $1 billion into the U.S. economy.

> On the hiring day in question, McDonald's and its franchisee operators ended up hiring 62,000 people. This was 24 percent more than planned.

Prior to its "National Hiring Day," McDonald's did some inspiring advertising. I was perusing *US* magazine, catching up on all the comings and goings of my favorite celebs, when I came across a full-page ad from McDonald's:

__We believe__
in quality.
We've believed in it
ever since we opened our first restaurant.
And we believe
that even though the word's gotten a little over-used by some,
it's more important to our business today than ever before.
For the meals we serve,
to the jobs we create.
That's why we offer people more than just jobs.
We offer them futures.
More than 50% of our franchisees started off behind the counter.
So did more than 75% of our restaurant managers
and many of our corporate staff.
So while you might think
that people just pass through,
the truth is that, increasingly, people who come here,
stay here and grow.
Something we believe makes this not just a better place to work.
but a better place all around.

Yes, it's advertising. I get that. It's meant to benefit the corporation. But it worked for me because it's inspiring. I like that it focuses on an often-misinterpreted or underreported fact. Today, fast food corporations employ large numbers of people, many of whom stay and thrive in that environment for a long time.

While the U.S. economy was still in the doldrums, the food service industry experienced fast growth in 2011, adding 63,500 additional jobs. According to the National Restaurant Association, it makes up 10 percent of America's workforce. In 2011, this represented 12.8 million people. By 2021, it's estimated this number will grow by 1.3 million.

McDonald's and the other fast food companies didn't always have so many restaurants and employ hundreds of thousands of people. Founded by individuals with limited capital but bold imaginations, they went from humble beginnings to revolutionize their industry. The pioneers who built these companies had a dream, and through hard work were able to achieve it.

The Early Days

Fast food, in one form or another, dates back to before the dawn of the 20th century. Prior to the Civil War, most American dining establishments were located at inns, boarding houses and taverns. Later, two very different restaurant types caught the public's fancy. Coffeehouses flourished as places where customers could socialize and engage in business. Oyster houses selling preserved oysters were also extremely popular. Both of these places allowed people to order on a "come and get it" basis instead of serving on a limited schedule.

In the 1830s, the Del-Monico family brought the restaurant concept to the forefront with several establishments they built in New York City. While Delmonico's catered to a rich clientele, other restaurants soon attracted the working class. Saloons were another place where light meals could be purchased, either free or cheaply (the drinks being the profit center). Many meals were sold around noontime, which became known as lunch. Food at these establishments could be eaten quickly and was ideal for those who had to hurry back to work.

Times continued to change and new quick-service restaurants emerged to cater to the growing customer base. In 1839, the first soda fountain was introduced in Philadelphia by Eugene Roussel. By the 1880s, many of the soda fountains, which had primarily sold carbonated beverages and ice cream sodas, began selling light food such as sandwiches. The addition of counters with customer seating gave birth to the luncheonette. Both the soda fountain and the luncheonette had a similar layout, a U-shaped counter where customers faced each other across from the kitchen. All of the restaurant operations—cooking and serving—were conducted inside the U-shaped counter.

From the luncheonette came the lunchroom and then the café. From there (taking a page from the factory assembly line) came the cafeteria. In 1885, the Exchange Buffet in New York City may have been the first restaurant to institute self-service. A unique offshoot of this concept was the automat. Customers selected food stored in six-by-eight-inch glass compartments placed along the walls of the automats. They put their money in the appropriate slot, opened the door of the compartment, and removed their food. It was the earliest form of a vending machine.

The restaurant industry underwent another renaissance with the widespread adoption of the automobile, which was introduced in the United States in the 1890s and became a major part of the American lifestyle by the 1950s. Restaurants continued to evolve to cater to the increasing numbers of customers in autos. In 1910, soda fountains instituted "curb service," in which the server would go out to the curb to take an order when a car pulled up, and then deliver the food on a tray.

Roadside stands also cropped up to accommodate the motorist. At their inception, the stands were set flush with the street or sidewalk, but as time went by, they were built set back from the roads to allow for parking. The majority of these were seasonal, since until the late 1920s most car travel occurred in warmer months. These roadside stands were called one of "America's last frontiers for independent businessmen." Entrepreneurs typically built the structures themselves, putting endless hard work and effort into their operations. In 1923, Frank Wright and Roy Allen opened the first A&W Root Beer stand in Sacramento, California. Food was brought out to customers sitting in their cars.

Out of the roadside stand came the drive-in and the highway coffee shop. After World War II, most drive-ins had a canopy under which autos parked and the carhops delivered the food. Before long, the drive-thru window (which had been introduced in California in the 1930s by Pig Stand Number 21) was commonplace. By the early 1950s, many drive-ins were adding "take home areas," "drive-up windows," and "indoor walk-ups" for customers who didn't want to eat in their cars. The fast food restaurant, as we know it, was born.

The Fast Food Pioneers

Although some depict the fast food chains as icy monoliths of corporate power, there's another perspective. Certainly, the big chains are just that, very large corporations far removed from the small start-up enterprises that they once were. Many of the pioneers who built them are gone today. But their visions, in many ways, still carry on.

Carl Karcher

In 1941, Carl and Margaret Karcher borrowed $311 against their car and, with another $15 they'd saved, bought a hot dog cart in Los Angeles. Their first-day sales totaled $14.75. Not quite five years later, they added three more carts and opened Carl's Drive-In Barbecue, which sold hamburgers among other food items. Today Carl's Jr. has more than 1,200 locations. It's part of CKE Restaurants, Inc., which includes Hardee's, La Salsa and Green Burrito.

Glen Bell

A hot dog cart also marked the entrepreneurial beginnings of Glen Bell, the founder of Taco Bell. In 1946, the 23-year-old marine veteran opened up his first hot dog cart in San Bernardino, California. He sold it in 1952 and began developing a restaurant that would sell both hamburgers and hot dogs. To differentiate himself from his competitors the McDonald brothers (Dick and Mac), who owned a nearby restaurant that also sold burgers, he elected to focus on a personal favorite: Mexican food.

In a strategic move, Bell opened his first restaurant in a predominately Hispanic area. He initially sold hot dogs and chili dogs with a homemade sauce that would eventually become the sauce for the store's tacos. When he was ready to introduce tacos at the restaurant, he sold them out of a side window for 19 cents apiece. They were an immediate success.

In 1951, Glenn Bell invented the preformed taco shell.

Bell opened up three Taco Tia stands in 1954 and 1955, but he had more ambitious plans. He sold the stands and used the proceeds to form a partnership with four Los Angeles Rams football players to open up another Mexican restaurant in Long Beach. They soon opened seven additional restaurants. Although they were successful, Bell still wanted to embark on a solo venture. He sold the chain to his partners, and in 1962, he opened the first Taco Bell in Downey, California. And the rest, as they say, is history.

In 1978, Bell sold his 868 Taco Bells to PepsiCo, Inc., making him millions of dollars. The company is now part of Yum! Brands, Inc., which also owns Pizza Hut and KFC. In 2010, Yum! Brands opened approximately four locations every day outside of the United States, helping to make it the world's largest fast food company. As of this writing, it has more than 37,000 restaurants in more than 117 countries. In February 2012, CEO David Novak said in a *USA Today* interview that over 70 percent of the company's profits were due to sales outside of the United States.

FAST FOOD VINDICATION

Harlan Sanders

Today, KFC operates more than 15,000 restaurants in more than 109 countries. They serve more than 12 million customers on a daily basis. Although it's now part of the Yum! Brands conglomerate, KFC had a less auspicious beginning.

In 1930, Harlan Sanders, the Colonel himself, opened his first restaurant, Sanders Court & Café, at the age of 40. This was after many years of holding down such various jobs as farm hand, army private, blacksmith's assistant, streetcar conductor, insurance salesman, railroad fireman, and operator of a service station in Corbin, Kentucky. Sanders Court & Café was part of the latter, and it was there that Sanders had his humble beginnings in the restaurant industry. He wore many hats in the operation, including chief cook, station operator and cashier. Seven years later, in 1939, a motel was added and the Sanders Court & Café grew to 142 seats. That same year, the pressure cooker was invented and Sanders began using it to fry chicken. A year after that, his famed original recipe was born.

In 1952, 22 years after opening Sanders Court & Café, Sanders started franchise efforts for his restaurant. He traveled from city to city, trying to interest franchisees by cooking and serving up his chicken recipe. By 1960, *at 70*, he'd realized his dream with more than 400 restaurants operated by 190 Kentucky Fried Chicken franchisees in the United States and Canada. In 2006, KFC served more than 1 billion chicken dinners in 80 countries.

"Colonel" Sanders not only epitomizes the success someone can achieve through determination and hard work, he's also proof that a person can fulfill his or her goal at any stage of life. In countries with an aging population, such as the United States, his path is an inspiring one. For him, it can be said that life began at 70.

Dave Thomas

Colonel Sanders helped another person overcome long odds to fulfill his dream: Dave Thomas, founder of Wendy's International, Inc. Born in 1932, Thomas was adopted when he was 6 weeks old.

When he was 5 years old, his adoptive mother died. He spent a number of years moving around the country with his adoptive father, who continually searched for employment during the Depression era.

Thomas began working at 12 as a counterperson in a Knoxville, Tennessee restaurant. At age 15, he dropped out of school while working at the Hobby House Restaurant in Fort Wayne, Indiana, at one point living at the YMCA after his family moved away. Sometime later, he met Harlan Sanders, one of his biggest influences. It so happened that his Hobby House boss also owned four money-losing Kentucky Fried Chicken restaurants. Thomas used his management expertise to bring the restaurants to profitability. Four years later, the restaurants were sold back to KFC. Thomas's percentage from the sale made him a millionaire at the age of 35.

In 1969, at age 37, Thomas opened the first Wendy's Old Fashioned Hamburgers Restaurant in Columbus, Ohio. Thirty-two years later, Wendy's opened its 6,000th restaurant.

Despite his great success, Thomas felt that dropping out of high school was the worst mistake he ever made. But he eventually did something about it. Forty-five years after leaving high school, he went to Coconut Creek High School in Fort Lauderdale, Florida, and earned his GED. He was named "Most Likely to Succeed" by the graduating class of 1993.

Fred DeLuca

When Fred DeLuca founded his restaurant chain, he'd already completed high school—but just barely. He was just 17 years old when, armed with a check from physicist (and family friend) Dr. Peter Buck, he opened his first submarine sandwich store. Nine years later, DeLuca and Buck had 16 restaurants in operation and were turning their attention to franchising their Subway stores. In late 2010, after being in business for 43 years, Subway bypassed McDonald's as the largest restaurant chain in the world with 33,749 locations worldwide.

Ray Kroc

McDonald's founder Ray Kroc was born in 1902. At the age of 15, he lied about his age so he could serve as a Red Cross ambulance driver in World War I, though the war ended before he could get to Europe. After a stint as a piano player, he became a paper cup salesman for the Lily-Tulip Cup Company and met Earl Prince, who had invented the five-spindled milk shake maker called the Multimixer.

Kroc was so impressed by the Multimixer's speed and efficiency that he took out a mortgage on his home and used all of his savings to become the device's exclusive distributor. For 17 years, he traveled all over the country selling it. In 1954, he noticed that Mac and Dick McDonald were generating such volume at their San Bernardino, California hamburger restaurant that they ran eight Multimixers simultaneously. Sensing an opportunity to sell more of his shake machines, he suggested that the McDonalds open several additional restaurants. When the brothers asked who would run the restaurants, Kroc thought about it and answered, "Well, what about me?" This was 1954 and Kroc was 52. His age and his sometimes-poor health didn't deter him from the hard work and long hours it took to grab his piece of the American dream. Looking back, he said, "I was 52 years old. I had diabetes and incipient arthritis. I had lost my gallbladder and most of my thyroid gland in earlier campaigns, but I was convinced that the best was ahead of me."

Kroc opened his first store in Des Plaines, Illinois, in 1955. First day's sales were $366.12. In 1961, he bought out the McDonald brothers and went on to achieve enormous global success. In early 2012, McDonald's had close to 14,000 locations in the United States. In total, the company operated around 33,000 restaurants worldwide, serving about 64 million people in 119 countries every day.

Ray Kroc died in 1984 at the age of 82. I didn't join the company until 1998 and never had the opportunity to meet him. But McDonald's Corporation still runs with the innovativeness, efficiency, cleanliness and core values that Kroc worked so hard to instill.

Fear of the American Dream

Before Ray Kroc had completed his second decade in the hamburger business, there were already strong feelings about his restaurants' dominance in the marketplace. In the 1970s, farm activist Jim Hightower voiced concern about the "McDonaldization of America." He believed the growing fast food industry would hurt smaller, independent businesses.

It's ironic that the fast food companies themselves started out as smaller, independent business enterprises. Is it a bad thing that the hardworking, self-sacrificing individuals who founded them were successful and grew their small businesses into larger ones? Do most mom-and-pop businesses want to remain small businesses and not grow and make more impact on their societies, their lives and their pocketbooks? Would it be fair to tell any entrepreneur that they shouldn't be too successful or grow too big? That wouldn't exactly be the American dream.

Growth and opportunity thrives at fast food corporations through their franchisees and the innovativeness of the people who work there. At McDonald's, it isn't uncommon to see husbands and wives, followed by their children, grab the entrepreneurial brass ring and become owner/operators of their own restaurants. Owner/operators bring with them creativity and innovativeness. The Egg McMuffin is among the menu items they've developed.

Hard work built the fast food restaurants where many of us eat today. Whether we like them or not, they're a vital part of the framework of our towns, cities, states and countries. And as we'll see, their impact is felt in ways far greater than the food they serve.

SEVEN

Work It!

"Without McDonald's, America Would Have Lost Jobs In May."

—Alex Goldmark writing for *Good Business* about the U.S. employment report for May 2011

Many common threads run through the origin stories of most of the fast food giants: the small beginnings, the risk-taking founders, an in-the-trenches ability to assess and meet the needs of their customers. Today, fast food corporations are major providers of employment opportunities in communities around the world. They're champions of diversity and offer attractive opportunities for advancement. Although there are bound to be unhappy and even disgruntled employees at these corporations, as at most companies, there are more than a few who actually enjoy working there. But for some reason there are people who refuse to believe this could be the case.

Anything but a Dead End Job

We've all heard the bad rap fast food employment gets: dead-end jobs at low wages. Douglas Coupland coined the word "McJob" in his novel *Generation X*, and it wasn't long before the word was defined in the Merriam-Webster's dictionary as "a low-paying job that requires little skill and provides little opportunity for advancement." But is this really true? If we take a closer look, there's much more than meets the eye.

Approximately 40 percent of the top 50 McDonald's executives started their careers by working in one of their company's restaurants. Over 50 percent of franchisees began as behind-the-counter crew. About 67,000 restaurant managers and assistant managers began as restaurant crew members. A large percentage of corporate operations employees also began as crew. As mentioned earlier, approximately one out of eight people in the United States has worked at McDonald's at some point in their lives. While many eventually leave to pursue other interests, it's obvious that some stay long-term and enjoy a great amount of success.

In 2000, while working in the real estate department in the McDonald's Southern California region, I attended a quarterly staff meeting. The general manager, Jeff Schwartz, asked approximately 100 people in the room to raise their hands if they had started with McDonald's as crew in a restaurant. Well over half the people put their hands in the air. It was amazing and inspiring that so many people who in high school worked behind the counter at a McDonald's were now in suits at a corporate staff meeting. This included Schwartz, who began cleaning bathrooms at McDonald's at age 15, then eventually went on to become CEO of McDonald's China operation until his retirement.

Karen King is another who began as a teenage crew member in a McDonald's restaurant and moved up through the ranks. In 2005, she became president of McDonald's East Division, an area that covered more than 5,000 restaurants. She credits her early experience as a crew member with lessons that still help in her career: "What McDonald's teaches its people are life skills. So I think about first jobs and paychecks, but also lessons about teamwork and self-confidence. For me, it was also about the opportunity to aspire to a career where the opportunities are limitless."

There are many other similar stories. Jeff Stratton, McDonald's executive vice president and chief restaurant officer, oversees the Restaurant Solutions Group (which impacts around 33,000 McDonald's restaurants worldwide). He began his career with McDonald's as a crewmember in Detroit in 1973 and climbed the ladder from there.

Tim Fenton, president of McDonald's Asia, Pacific, Middle East and Africa, also began as a crewmember. So did Janice L. Fields, president of McDonald's USA, and Steve Plotkin, West Division president for McDonald's USA. Jim Skinner, retired vice chairman and chief executive officer joined the company in 1971 as a restaurant manager trainee after serving almost ten years in the U.S. Navy. And there are many more.

So it's obvious the dictionary definition of "McJob" isn't an accurate one, either in the U.S. or overseas. A recent study by Leeds Metropolitan University in the United Kingdom found that "McDonald's approach to recruitment, training and development allowed employees to progress." Eight out of 10 employees thought of the McDonald's job as a long-term career. In addition, 83 percent of the employees said they had either developed or improved their skills, and 96 percent said they thought these skills would help them with future employers.

While many critics have no firsthand knowledge of what it's like to work at McDonald's or other fast food restaurants, the enterprising university professor Jerry Newman decided to find out what actually happens behind the counter. Researching his 2007 book *My Secret*

Life on the McJob, he worked "undercover" at seven different fast food restaurants over a 14-month period. While his primary purpose was to assess the management styles of the various supervisors at the restaurants, he found out something very interesting along the way, especially if you consider fast food work easy and non-challenging. "I'm living testament that this job is hard," he wrote.

McDonald's Corporation also offers computerized English language classes and other educational opportunities crew members can take advantage of on their breaks or after work. In addition, employees at company-owned restaurants can participate in 401(k) retirement accounts matched by company contributions.

Fortune magazine has named McDonald's as the "Best Place to Work for Minorities." According to *Fortune*, in order to be named to this list, a company must "make an effort not only to hire minorities, but also to retain them and promote them through the ranks. [McDonald's] actively interacts with outside minority communities and makes management accountable for diversity efforts."

Gerry Fernandez, the president of the MultiCultural Foodservice & Hospitality Alliance, said, "Seeing McDonald's being named as the top company for minorities by *Fortune* magazine is no surprise to those of us in the food service industry. McDonald's continues to set even higher standards for themselves and do more to promote diversity and inclusion across the entire hospitality industry." This includes top-ranking executives like CEO Don Thompson, an African American, and Executive Vice President, General Counsel Gloria Santona, a Latina.

Training, Development and Upward Mobility

McDonald's spends more than $1 million each year training its employees. Its well-regarded education center, Hamburger University, in Oak Brook, Illinois, hosts over 5,000 students each year. The 130,000-square-foot facility has 13 classrooms, a 300 seat auditorium, 3 kitchen labs and several training labs. There are also 22 regional training teams throughout the United States, and

Hamburger Universities now operate in Munich, London, Sydney, Hong Kong, Tokyo and Brazil. Over the years, more than 275,000 people worldwide have "graduated" from Hamburger University. This includes over 80,000 restaurant managers, franchisees and middle management. It also includes me.

The quality of McDonald's training is such that it's the only fast food restaurant education that's been deemed eligible for college credits through the American Council on Education. In Britain, McDonald's was recently approved to offer Level 3 courses, which allows students to combine in-house classes with others to qualify for the standard A-levels or advanced diplomas. Then-Prime Minister Gordon Brown praised the new program by stating, "I think that is the important thing, companies prepared to train people up which they weren't doing before, in the way that we want them to do, in a far greater number, so that people have the qualifications for the future."

McDonald's also provides e-learning to its employees. These are computer courses designed in such a way that employees can learn at their own pace. Classroom courses are available that can help enable crew members advance to restaurant management positions and even higher. Qualifying employees receive up to $5,250 per year for classes that will benefit them in present or future positions. And each year, McDonald's gives 52 scholarships to their restaurant employees in the United States through its National Employee Scholarship Program.

McDonald's isn't the only fast food company to beat the "dead-end job" rap. Eunice Allotey, a single mother of two, took a job at a Detroit Kentucky Fried Chicken in 1982, shortly after immigrating to the U.S. from Ghana in West Africa. She started behind the counter for minimum wage, but within a few years, she worked herself up to the position of operations coach for KFC's Detroit region, overseeing 53 restaurants. Her annual base salary in the '80s was $100,000 plus up to 25 percent more in bonuses, depending on individual and company performance. Not too shabby.

> KFC recently announced it would offer the opportunity for its staff in Britain to take a three-year course in business studies while working full-time. Upon graduation, the employees would be eligible for area manager positions and jobs working in the corporate office.

So when Eric Schlosser and Charles Wilson assert in their book *Chew on This* that "a McJob is a job that doesn't promise much of a future," this is clearly not always the case. Dr. Jerry Newman agrees. After his undercover stint working at seven fast food restaurants, he said, "I've found many bright, hardworking people working in fast food…Those workers who had aspirations to learn and advance were duly rewarded. Not only was there an opportunity to build new skills in fast food, there was an expectation that this would happen."

Compensation

As in many industries, entry-level jobs in the fast food business generally pay near the minimum wage. Effective July 24, 2008, the Federal minimum wage in the United States was $6.55 per hour. In 2007, the U.S. Department of Labor listed the median hourly wage for fast food cooks at $7.75 per hour. By comparison, gaming dealers were listed as earning $7.51 and ushers, lobby attendants and ticket takers earned a median hourly wage of $7.85.

Job Satisfaction Is in the Eye of the Beholder

It's true that most fast food workers don't parlay their positions into lifelong careers. The jobs often provide what a person is looking for at that particular time of their life: a high school student with cash for a car, a college student with tuition payments, or a senior citizen with an income supplement or an opportunity for social interaction. Fast food jobs attract people of all ages, races and genders. Many of the people who seek this kind of employment get exactly what they're looking for. Some move on to successful careers outside the fast food industry, such as talk show host Jay Leno, Amazon.com founder and CEO Jeff Bezos, Olympic gold medal winner Carl Lewis, former Indiana Governor Joe Kernan and former Snap-On Tools CEO Robert Cornog. All are former McDonald's employees.

Everyone who works at these jobs receives training for such things as efficiency, proper sanitation and safe food handling procedures and good customer service skills. Teamwork and professional behavior are valued and fostered. Bilingual workers are also appreciated. Those who exhibit strong skills in these areas are often given the opportunity for further training and promotion.

When the economy is in turmoil, more people look for part-time jobs to help make ends meet. Many businesses, large and small, have folded in recent years, cutting back positions or going out of business entirely. When the economy sinks, the large fast food corporations typically still stand strong, providing low-cost meals and employment opportunities for those in need of a steady paycheck. If they didn't exist, there would be fewer places for people to turn for work. Recently, McDonald's even joined forces with a government-run British job placement service to provide work trials for the long-time unemployed at McDonald's restaurants throughout the UK.

The Fast Food Workforce

So who are the workers behind the counters at fast food restaurants? Why do they work there? The fast food workforce is diverse, but the media's focus has largely been restricted to the teenage worker. Critics of the fast food industry often point to the plight of the poor teenager who toils away at the dead-end fast food job. But is that really the case?

The Teenage Worker

Teenagers choose to work for a variety of reasons, but we all know spending money is a chief motivator. A recent study found that approximately 54 percent of American teens don't get an allowance from their parents. In 2005, the U.S. Department of Labor reported that 50 percent of the youths in America had informal jobs, like yard work or babysitting, by as early as 12 years of age. At one time, teenagers accounted for 70 percent of the newspaper carriers in the United States. By the time they reach 15 years old, almost two-thirds of teens are employed in some capacity. Employment has many benefits for teens. Learning to work with a team, taking responsibility, mastering new tasks, personal hygiene and professional behavior are just a few. Increased self-esteem, feelings of independence and competence, and learning time and money management are also important. Teens who work a limited number of hours are more apt to have a job after completing high school and are also more likely to earn more money upon graduation.

The shortage of teenage labor impacts the fast food industry. In the 1990s approximately 45 percent of McDonald's U.S. restaurant crew was under age 20. In 2007, they only accounted for 33 percent. About 50 percent of fast food restaurant employees today are between the ages of 16 and 25. However, while the number of jobs in the fast food industry is predicted to increase approximately 17 percent by 2020, the number of workers between 16 and 25 is likely to rise only by 0.3 percent.

The Older Worker

A group has emerged that helps fill the void left by the declining number of working teens: the senior adult. In 1999, approximately 3 percent of the U.S. working population (about 4 million people) was 65 or older. This number rose to 14.5 percent by 2006 and is projected to reach 19.7 percent by 2014.

The rise in senior workers is due to many causes. First, we're living longer and healthier, and some of us don't want to stop working at the traditional retirement age. A 2006 MetLife Mature Market Institute report found that of the 66- to 70- year-olds surveyed, 72 percent worked because they liked to be "active and engaged." Forty-two percent cited social interaction as an incentive. Other reasons include financial and health benefits, avoiding depression and loneliness, and for a sense of purpose.

A May 2007 article in *The Fresno Bee* told the story of Dorothy Evans, a 92-year-old former restaurant owner who worked at a McDonald's restaurant in California 20 hours a week. She joined the company in 1993, starting as a dining-room hostess, then preparing desserts, salads and french fries. She enjoyed the money and feeling productive. "I don't do very good just sitting around," she said. "I have always said that rocking chairs cause people to get old. And I don't want that to be me."

As early as 1986, McDonald's made an effort to target older workers through the McMasters program instituted in Baltimore. Franchise operators in the Baltimore area worked with local government agencies charged with helping older people find jobs. The success of the program benefited McDonald's—senior workers are generally dependable, saving the company money through reduced turnover costs. But it also benefited the rapidly growing older worker population. And what better inspiration for them than Ray Kroc, who didn't even open his first McDonald's until he was in his mid-50s?

KFC also implemented a senior employment program called "Colonel's Tradition" that places recruitment flyers in its restaurants to target senior adults. These flyers read, "Come join our tradition—started by the Colonel when he was age 65." Like Ray Kroc, Colonel Sanders is an inspiration to the older employee. He kept working until he was 90.

The Physically or Mentally Challenged Worker

The fast food industry also employs those who are mentally and physically challenged. McDonald's created McJOBS, a program that has been in place for over 20 years to employ and train mentally and physically challenged individuals "They are people who need work, and we need people to work," said Mark Brownstein, a McDonald's owner/operator in Orange County, California. "You wonder why everybody makes a big deal about it." Another McDonald's franchisee, Jonah Kaufman, employed 26 challenged employees (mostly with Down syndrome) at his stores in Long Island. The key, he said, is "to try not to treat them differently." Other fast food companies also have been supportive of working with this special class of worker. As early as the 1980s, Carl's Jr. started using a Braille keyboard that could be overlaid on the point-of-purchase computer terminals. McDonald's also has used Braille and sign language for deaf workers.

The Non-College Degree Worker

Another group that benefits from fast food employment is those who opt to enter the workforce full-time after high school instead of seeking college educations. This is a large percentage of the U.S. population. While 64 percent of high school graduates attend college, only 29 percent of Americans aged 25 to 29 hold bachelor degrees. In addition, only one out of four students in degree programs at two-year colleges actually ends up getting a degree or certificate.

There are many factors that prevent a young adult from attending or finishing college. The reality is some simply don't have the academic skills to finish. Others may not have the money, drive, self-discipline, or maturity. Some may have family circumstances or health issues that get in the way. Regardless of the reasons, there are many career paths that are beyond the reach of the majority of those without college educations. These people still need to support themselves and perhaps their families. So what do they do? They take advantage of many career opportunities that don't require a degree— like the fast food industry, where hard work, drive and determination can lead to great success.

The Unusual Worker

People work for a variety of reasons, and sometimes it's just because they genuinely like their job and appreciate their employer. Luke Pittard, a McDonald's employee in Wales, was one man who really loved his job. He won the lottery and did what a lot of people would do in his circumstances—he quit his position training employees at McDonald's. But he missed it, and eighteen months later he went back to work there, making less money than he received from the *interest* on his lottery winnings. "Everyone thinks I'm [crazy], but I tell them there's more to life than money," he said. "I loved working at McDonald's before I became a millionaire, and I'm really enjoying being back there again."

The Diverse Workforce

The fast food industry is a champion of diversity. Subway is one of many examples of this. About 34 percent of its franchisees are women. Approximately 24 percent are minorities. Around 10 percent of Subway franchisees are 62 or older, and close to 30 percent of franchisees employ people 62 and older. Almost 80 percent of Subway franchisees employ ethnic minorities.

Among other diversity recognitions, Yum! Brands has been named one of the "30 Best Companies for Diversity" by *Black Enterprise* magazine and has made *Fortune* magazine's "Best Companies for Minorities" list several consecutive years. Burger King has maintained a Diversity Action Council (DAC) advisory board since 1991, with members including Burger King employees and others from outside the company. The DAC represents the community and franchise interests of Asian Americans, African Americans, Hispanics and other minority groups.

McDonald's Corporation "treats diversity as an initiative rather than a program," according to Pat Harris, its global chief diversity officer. Formal diversity efforts, a business objective for the company, began in the late 1970s. Today, over 55 percent of McDonald's employees throughout the United States are of a racial or ethnic minority. Approximately 61 percent are females. In addition, over 40 percent of its U.S. franchisees are women and minorities.

University professor Jerry Newman, who studied the culture of fast food during his time spent in various restaurants, sums it up well: "Do fast food restaurants discriminate? The answer is an emphatic

'NO!' I saw people of every nationality in my seven jobs. Stores are populated by males and females, older workers and younger workers. The promotion pipeline also was charged with the right mix of people. Over the years, I've consulted with hundreds of companies, and none of them could boast a better mix of genders, ages, and nationalities than I saw across the seven stores."

The fast food giants have led the way in their focus on diversity, education, and employee growth opportunities. And the industry's positive contributions don't end with their employees. As we'll see, they extend from their backyards to around the world.

EIGHT

Good Neighbor Policy

"If you are going to take money out of a community,

give something back."

—Ray Kroc, founder of McDonald's Corporation

We've seen how some have singled out the fast food chains for their perceived roles in the obesity epidemic and the quality of their jobs. But surely even the detractors will admit these corporations are charitable, with well-known philanthropic efforts benefiting local communities, the nation and the world. Most, if not all, of these fast food corporations give back in a variety of areas. They donate money and time to such causes as hunger, education, troubled and endangered children, medical research, child adoption, emergency efforts and many other worthwhile causes.

And yet the critics are loathe to acknowledge this philanthropy. On mcspotlight.org, for example, one vented: "McDonald's are [sic] of course simply a particularly arrogant, shiny and self-important example of a system which values profits at the expense of anything else."

First, a reality check. All "for-profit" businesses, small to large, are in business to make money. That's a given. But it doesn't mean they care about making a profit over *anything else*. If that were the case, they wouldn't pour millions of dollars into philanthropic efforts. To be sure, there is publicity value and good will to be gained from charitable activities, but much of their good works are done outside the spotlight.

If we take a look at a few of the most important issues of the day, we're likely to find one or more of the fast food chains involved in related charitable causes.

Adoption

Children are a big part of the philanthropic efforts embraced by fast food corporations. One of the most admirable was started by Dave Thomas of Wendy's. As a child of adoption, Thomas felt very strongly about helping children who were waiting to be adopted. He worked through the years to help bring these children together with loving adoptive parents and families.

In 1990, at the request of President George H. W. Bush, Thomas took the lead of the White House Initiative on Adoption. Among other things, he launched a letter-writing campaign to Fortune 1,000 CEOs to give adoption benefits to their employees. He also asked state governors to do the same for state employees. He continued his work with President Bill Clinton, who in 1996 signed the Tax Credit Bill, which gave a one-time tax credit of $5,000 to parents when they adopted. Clinton also signed the Adoption and Safe

Families Act, which lessened the waiting time for kids in foster care, making the adoption process faster and providing for state incentives and accountability.

In 1992, Thomas created the Dave Thomas Foundation for Adoption, which gives grants to regional and national adoption agencies for programs that increase awareness and help make adoption easier and affordable. The goal is to significantly increase the adoption rate among the 150,000-plus children in foster care available for adoption in North America.

One of the foundation's programs is Wendy's Wonderful Kids. It uses money raised from Wendy's restaurants, customers and other partners to help local adoption agencies hire recruiters solely focused on placing children in foster care with adoptive parents. They began with seven recruiters and quickly expanded to 105 in all 50 states, the District of Columbia and Canada. As of late April 2011, the program had a total of 6,864 children, with 4,376 matched, 690 in pre-adoptive homes and 2,160 children adopted.

Healthcare and Support

Dave Thomas's charitable efforts weren't limited to adoption-related causes. Among other things, he contributed millions of dollars to medical centers including Nationwide Children's Hospital in Columbus, Ohio, where he created the Dave Thomas Family Primary Care Center and the Dave and Lorraine Thomas Clinical Laboratory. Through a $2 million contribution, the R. David Thomas Outpatient Chemotherapy Center was established at the Arthur G. James Cancer Hospital at Ohio State University.

McDonald's also contributes to the health of children all over the world. Since 1984, McDonald Corporation's "charity of choice" has been Ronald McDonald House Charities (RMHC), a non-profit organization that helps families and children in 52 countries. Ronald McDonald House is a "home away from home" for families of kids receiving care at nearby hospitals. Currently, there are more than 300 such houses around the world. Each can accommodate approximately 15 families, costing them each $5 to $15 dollars a day—but only if the families can afford to pay. Ronald McDonald Family Room provides rooms inside hospitals near intensive care and pediatric units for families to sit, relax, or have a meal. The Ronald McDonald Care Mobile provides cost-effective medical, dental and health education to children who are underserved in urban and rural areas around the world.

Another way McDonald's Corporation supports RMHC is through its World Children's Day. This annual event of fundraising in the individual restaurants is a joint effort between local McDonald's offices and employees, its owner/operators, customers and suppliers around the world. Since its 2002 inception, World Children's Day has raised hundreds of millions of dollars. The organization hoped to raise $600 million by the year-end 2011 to build 68 new Ronald McDonald's Houses, open 56 additional Ronald McDonald Family Rooms and add 23 more Ronald McDonald Care Mobiles to the existing fleet. This fleet would allow them to provide medical and dental care to more than 420,000 kids annually. At the end of 2011, there were 44 McDonald's Care Mobiles.

> In mid-2011, RMHC had 30,000-plus volunteers ranging from age 9 to 92.

Ronald McDonald House Charities helps more than 10,000 people every day and more than 3.6 million families each year. As of 2006, approximately 10 million families had stayed at a Ronald McDonald House, taking advantage of the more than 6,000 rooms available on a nightly basis around the world. In 2007, 73 percent of top-ranked children's hospitals in the U.S. and abroad benefited from at least one of the core programs of the charity.

"People don't realize when you have a sick child, you don't care about cooking a meal, you don't care about shopping, you don't care about anything but being at hospital 24/7," said Cheryl Klee, who used the Ronald McDonald house in Bismarck, North Dakota many times since it opened in 1992. Another parent, Maria Ponce, stayed at the Ronald McDonald House in Galveston, Texas, after her child was born prematurely. "If not for this house, I could not be with my son," she said. "And it is not only me—everyone needs this... This is like a home with everything you need. Plus you are around people who care and have experience. I am so grateful. This is like a second home, but better."

Some families who have benefited from stays at these houses later give back to the organization. "The Ronald McDonald House was such a blessing to our family during such a traumatic time in our lives," said Dawn Pridgen, a mother of twins born 13 weeks premature in Tifton, Georgia. "The RMH provided us a place to stay, home-cooked meals by volunteers every night and interactions with other families that were experiencing the same emotions that we were." They stayed at the Ronald McDonald House in Macon for 101 days. Five years later, Dawn and her husband, Shane, were involved in a benefit fundraiser for the house.

Those who help bring Ronald McDonald Houses to their local areas also speak of them as a place where visitors can feel instantly at home. When Tony Diez and Keith Swarts were working to get a Ronald McDonald House in Omaha, they visited an existing one in Kansas City. "We could smell spaghetti cooking on the stove," Diez said. "That's when we knew that Ronald McDonald Houses are really home." Swarts echoed a common refrain among RMH organizers when he said, "This is probably one of my greatest projects because of the families we've helped. We didn't have enough places for families to stay and had had a family sleeping in their car in the parking garage. I'll always remember the day we opened the Ronald McDonald House and families moved in."

> Edgar Dworsky of ConsumerWorld.org recently complained that McDonald's was less than upfront about the amount of money from the sale of Happy Meals that it donates to RMHC (one penny per meal). He said that McDonald's was not open about the small percentage of its contribution, although it's clearly mentioned in its advertising. McDonald's responded to this criticism by stating that this contribution "translates to millions of dollars raised each year given the millions of Happy Meals we sell each year – a little can add up to make a big change."

Yum! Restaurants International also works in several countries to help children and fund clinical research. Their Millennium Foundation raises money for medical studies at one of Australia's largest teaching hospitals. Their Reach program, also in Australia, works to help reduce youth suicide through peer support groups and the teaching of life skills. And KFC in the United Kingdom supports ChildLine, a no-cost 24-hour help line for children and adolescents facing crises.

Education

Most fast food corporations also encourage and foster education programs. Across the United States, budget cutbacks have resulted in increased class sizes and many programs being cut from the curriculum. One of the most alarming statistics is the dropout rate: One out of four U.S. high school students leaves before getting a diploma. Also, one out of three minority students drops out. Several fast food corporations have instituted efforts to help reverse this trend.

McDonald's has reached out to adolescents and teens with several education initiatives. One such program is All American Achievers, rolled out in 2008 to showcase top-performing seventh and eighth grade students and encourage community service and character development. In addition, high school seniors can receive college scholarships through RMHC. Over $29 million in scholarship money has been given to date through four different scholarship programs: Hispanic American Commitment to Educational Resources, Asian Students Increasing Achievement, RMCH Scholars, and RMHC African American Future Achievers.

McDonald's also fosters education around the world. In Australia, McDonald's Camp Quality Puppet Program has reached more than 2.5 million children at approximately 8,500 schools with a puppet show about cancer's effects and treatments. McDonald's also sponsored the Sue the Dinosaur exhibition at the Field Museum in Chicago, as well as the cast replication of Sue that's travelled across the U.S., Japan and China. Other education programs provided by McDonald's throughout the world include:

- Fire Prevention Program (Russia)—Focusing on fire safety and prevention, this program has reached more than 31,000 children.
- Seat Belt Safety Program (New Zealand)—Through the Ronald McDonald show "Make It Click," more than 84,000 students in more than 800 schools have been taught the importance of seat belts and road safety.
- Ronald Sports Program (Netherlands)—More than 355,000 kids have taken part in the Ronald Sport and Active Shows.

Taco Bell also helps kids through their partnership with Boys & Girls Clubs of America. Since 1995, they've reached more than 1 million teenagers a year, with over $17 million from franchisees and customers going toward educational, leadership and career opportunities. Another Yum! Brand, Pizza Hut, has the BOOK IT! and BOOK IT! Beginners programs. With the goal of developing a child's love of reading, Pizza Hut has been reaching kindergarteners through books since 1985. KFC offers scholarships for teenagers with financial needs through its Colonel's Scholars program, which gives up to $20,000 to high school seniors who want to attend a public in-state college or university.

Actor Mark Wahlberg and the Taco Bell Foundation for Teens worked together in 2010 and 2011 on the Graduate to Go program, which raises money to help teens learn the importance of staying in school and getting a high school diploma. Wahlberg continues to be an ambassador for the program.

Yum! Brands also provides education initiatives around the world. In China, KFC and the China Youth Development Foundation created the KFC China First Light Foundation to provide scholarships to students at universities and colleges in cities such as Guangzhou, Tianjin, Wuhan, Shenzhen and Chengdu. KFC China will also give part-time jobs at their restaurants to students. KFC-Pizza Hut in Thailand has instituted the We Do Society Right program, in which money collected at Pizza Hut and KFC in Thailand has been used to build 10 elementary schools since the year 2000, as well as provide books, clothes, tables and chairs, scholarships and medicine packages. In addition, the KFC Victoria White Lion Program in Australia gives vocational training to teenagers who have been through the juvenile justice system.

Dave Thomas of Wendy's also believed in education, particularly since he so regretted dropping out of high school. He established Duke University's Thomas Center, home to the Fuqua School of Business Executive Education programs. He was one of the founders of the private Wellington School in Columbus, Ohio, and supported the Enterprise Ambassador Program at Nova University in South Florida, which familiarizes high school students with the free enterprise system through a mentoring program and classes.

Burger King also champions education through its Scholars Program. Open to high school seniors in the United States, Canada and Puerto Rico, this program gives $1,000 cash awards to be used toward educational expenses in the first year of college or postsecondary vocational or technical school. Since its inception in 2000, the program has awarded over $10 million in scholarships. And Burger King's Have It Your Way Foundation and Burger King/McLamore Foundation honor students who demonstrate efforts in community service and scholastic achievement.

World Hunger

Another important issue addressed by fast food corporations is hunger or food insecurity. The World Food Summit of 1996 defined food security as existing only when all people at all times have "sustainable physical or economic access to enough safe, nutritious, and socially acceptable food for a healthy and productive life." In 2009, around 50.2 million people in the United States lived in food-insecure homes. Today approximately 12 million children in America are at risk for going hungry. Yum! Brands is one of many organizations dedicated to combating hunger. Their YUMeals program, now the largest prepared-food donation program in the world, donates food to more than 2,000 hunger relief organizations across the country, benefiting many needy families.

More than 850 million people in the world today are starving, and Yum! Brands also battles hunger on the global stage. To help raise money, create awareness and inspire people to volunteer, they launched the first annual World Hunger Relief Week in 2007. Almost 1 million Yum! Brands employees, franchisees and their families worked 4 million volunteer hours and raised $16 million for the United Nations World Food Programme and other hunger relief agencies. It was one of the largest coordinated volunteer efforts in history.

Disaster Relief

Unexpected calamity tests us as a society, and it's inspiring to see how many put their personal interests aside and do everything in their power to help make things right. This includes fast food corporations, which have done much in these times of great need.

On September 11, 2001, America was shocked by an act of terrorism so horrible it still resonates deeply today. We watched with pride as approximately 40,000 rescue workers toiled away, doing everything they could to find the living and the dead. McDonald's stepped up and did their part, providing more than 750,000 free meals to rescue workers at the World Trade Center and the Pentagon.

McDonald's has also been quick to provide monetary assistance when natural disasters strike. The company raised $9.8 million for Hurricane Katrina relief efforts, and dispensed $300,000 in emergency loans to employees who were displaced by the hurricane. It also gave Happy Meal toys to kids residing in shelters. When the 2004 tsunami hit Southeast Asia, McDonald's and RMHC raised approximately $3.3 million in relief funds in the first month after the disaster. In the first week after the 2008 earthquake in Sichuan, China, McDonald's China and Ronald McDonald House Charities of China committed $1.5 million RMB to relief efforts. In addition, they provided 22,000 meals to relief workers, military, police and fire department workers, as well as to hospitals that were running out of food. They also helped support local blood drive efforts by setting up food and beverage stations at the donation centers and offering free meal incentives through in-store promotions.

Community Efforts

Fast food industry philanthropic efforts are felt almost daily on the community level. Local youth athletic teams, schools and even dietetic associations have benefited from donations. McDonald's employees are given the opportunity to spend a workday volunteering for an agency or charity of their choice on Ray Kroc's birthday every year. I was one of these employees who gave my time, helping out at a school for the profoundly disabled. Working with those young people was a life-changing experience and I hope that I helped them in at least some small way. I consider myself a charitable person, but I have to admit that if McDonald's hadn't encouraged me and all of its employees to volunteer their time, I probably wouldn't have gone there. I'm so glad I did.

In a 2001 *Time* magazine article titled "America's Hamburger Helper," Edwin M. Reingold wrote of the aftermath of the riots in South Central Los Angeles in which hundreds of businesses had been destroyed by fire. Amazingly, not one McDonald's restaurant had been burned, which allowed them to open their doors to feed the police, firefighters, National Guard and the public at large. They also delivered free lunches to 300 students at St. Thomas Aquinas Elementary School, which couldn't cook with its utilities down.

Reingold summed it up well: "McDonald's stands out not only as one of the more socially responsible companies in America but also as one of the nation's few truly effective social engineers. Both its franchise operators, who own 83 percent of all McDonald's restaurants, and company officials sit on boards of local and national minority service organizations, allowing the company to claim that its total involvement in everything from the Urban League and the NAACP to the U.S. Hispanic Chamber of Commerce may constitute the biggest volunteer program of any business in the nation."

So when people knock large corporations and claim they lack a human side, that's not always the case. McDonald's founder Ray Kroc set the best example with his belief that the corporation, including its employees and franchisees, should also be in the business of community service and helping others. Many years after his death, this practice continues, and the same also can be said of the fast food industry in general.

NINE

Bigger Isn't Always Better

"Entrées at family-style eateries posted 271 more calories,
435 more milligrams of sodium and 16 more grams of fat
than fast-food restaurants."

—Helen Wu, assistant policy analyst at Rand
Corporation, on a recent study

Whether at fast food restaurants, sit-down restaurants, or at home, we can eat more calories than we should each day in a single meal. If it's just a day here and there, it's not likely a problem. If it's a lot of days, there's room for change.

I've spoken to many people who are trying to lose weight, and many don't actually know their recommended daily calorie level. This is important information, not only to maintain existing weight but to lose pounds, if needed. Do you know what your maintenance calories are? How about a recommended calorie count to lose weight or even to gain weight, if that's your goal? It varies from person to person. One number doesn't work for all.

If you don't know your appropriate daily calorie intake level, you're not alone. I deal with this every day. Let's look at Soso Whaley's case. At the time she embarked on her McDonald's-only diet, she was 49 years old, five feet, three inches tall, and weighed 175 pounds. This equates to a BMI of 31, which is considered obese. So, she started out at an unhealthy weight, perhaps due to overeating on a consistent basis and lack of regular exercise. She says she limited herself to 1,800 to 2,000 calories during her diet. On "days off," she had more than that. She also engaged in moderate exercise for approximately one hour about three times a week.

Whaley lost weight because the calories she consumed during her McDonald's-only diet were less than what she normally ate. But had she weighed less (that is, in the recommended BMI range), this wouldn't necessarily have been the case.

A healthy BMI for Whaley would be less than 25, but over 18.5. To land at the top of this recommended range (24.9), she would need to weigh 140 pounds. Remember, she was at 175 pounds, which wasn't a healthy weight for her. To maintain a weight of 140 pounds, with moderate exercise and keeping her age at 49 for purposes of this discussion, she would need to consume about 1,800 calories. At this healthier weight, this amount of calories probably wouldn't result in weight loss. If she wanted to lose weight with a goal of achieving a BMI of 23, she would need to cut 500 calories a day, for a weight loss of one pound a week, until she lost ten more pounds. That isn't 1,800 calories per day for weight loss. It's more like 1,300 calories.

Whaley went on an extremely restricted diet in which she ate all of her meals at one restaurant. This is no way to eat for life, nor something I recommend. But the fact remains that she did lose weight. She did this by (a) eating fewer calories than she normally did, and (b) engaging in physical activity. This is key. Burning calories through exercise while simultaneously cutting the amount of calories normally consumed should lead to weight loss. It's a simple strategy that forms the basis of most weight-loss programs.

I work with many people who are unable to lose weight, even though they are eating less and exercising more. They're confused, stymied and more than a little frustrated. I can certainly understand their concern. In trying to determine where these individuals might make some changes, I delve deeper into their eating habits. I often arrive at the same conclusion—they are still eating too much. They're usually shocked to hear it. And that's *before* I tell them how many calories they should consume in a day.

The Mifflin-St Jeor equation is considered to be the best indicator of determining maintenance and weight-loss calories. It involves a bit of math, but it's well worth pulling out the calculator.

To determine your basal metabolic rate (BMR), which is the amount of calories your body burns on its own without movement/exercise, please calculate the following:

Men: (10 x weight in kg) + (6.25 x height in centimeters) – (5 x age in years) +5

Women: (10 x weight in kg) + (6.25 x height in centimeters) – (5 x age in years) – 161

To add in calories for you particular exercise level, multiply the BMR number calculated above by the appropriate number below:

cont. on page 112

cont. from page 111

If sedentary (little to no exercise, a job that isn't active): 1.2
Light activity (light exercise one to three days a week): 1.375
Moderate activity (moderate exercise three to five days a week): 1.55
Very active (intense exercise six to seven days a week): 1.725
Extreme activity (very intense exercise, a job that's physically demanding): 1.9

To lose one pound a week, you need to reduce this number by 500 calosries. It isn't recommended to eat less than 1200 calories a day without medical supervision.

Note:
To determine your weight in kg, take your weight in pounds and divide it by 2.2.

To determine your height in centimeters, multiply your height in inches by 2.54.

I Can't Believe I Ate the Whole Thing!

In the past twenty years or so, the portion sizes of foods eaten in America have increased dramatically. In a University of North Carolina study, researchers found that, on average, the typical American eats more at every meal compared to twenty years ago. Between 1971 and 2000, the average daily calorie intake increased by approximately 335 calories for females and 168 calories for males. While many point their finger squarely at fast food as the cause, the study found we're eating too much at a variety of places, including conventional sit-down restaurants and our homes. And most of us are doing this without even realizing it. Just about everything is bigger, and where nutrition is concerned, that isn't usually better.

Over the years, the average size of bagels increased from three inches in diameter to six inches. This added over 200 calories. For us moviegoers, the size of theater popcorn increased from five cups (around 270 calories) to 11 cups (around 630 calories). These are just two examples from a mile-long list.

Americans are dining out more than ever. We can eat too much at home, to be sure, but we can eat too much outside the house too. This can occur in all kinds of restaurants, from fast food to fine dining.

Today the average American spends close to 50 percent of every food dollar on food eaten outside the home. According to the National Restaurant Association, this number was only 25 percent in 1950. Studies have shown that men eat away from home more than women. But changes in eating habits have occurred across the board. The University of North Carolina study found that between 1977 and 1996, the number of Americans 19 to 39 who had eaten outside the home on any particular day had doubled.

An 18-month study by the Rand Corporation found that 96% of entrées sold at chain restaurants in the United States exceeded the recommended daily limits for calories, total fat, saturated fat and sodium. The study looked at the nutritional value of 30,923 items from 245 restaurants located throughout the U.S. Some of the findings were:
- Appetizers at sit-down restaurants had more calories (average 813) than entrées (average 674).
- Entrées at sit-down family-style restaurants had more calories, fat and sodium on average than meals at fast food restaurants.
- Shakes and floats marketed to kids often had more calories than regular menu drinks, which had a median of 360 calories.

FAST FOOD VINDICATION

Americans are snacking more than ever, with snack calories doubling between the 1970s and the 1990s. Some may be surprised to learn that most of these extra calories *weren't* consumed at fast food restaurants. Men consumed only eight additional snack calories and women ate only six more snack calories daily at fast food restaurants during this period. And Dr. Alanna Moshfegh of the U.S. Department of Agriculture found sweeteners and desserts jointly accounting for nearly a quarter of the daily calorie intake of children. These can come from a variety of places—from a convenience store to Mom's home-baked cookies to a local eatery.

> Recently the phone rang in my house and my husband picked it up. I was unloading groceries at the time and an unopened bag of walnuts was sitting on the counter. He opened it and started munching. By the time his telephone conversation was over, the bag was empty. He'd eaten every last walnut, for a total of about 2,000 calories. This is the amount of calories he should have in an entire day, not for a snack.

Many of the people I speak with patronize fast food restaurants. How often and what they consume varies, but they eat there all the same. It's rare for me to talk to a group in which not even one person ever eats at a fast food restaurant. Only once—when I was teaching a class on heart health and lowering cholesterol levels—have I talked to a group in which each attendee said they didn't indulge in fast food.

Yet the majority of the attendees were overweight or obese. So I inquired about their eating habits to try and figure out what caused their weights to be outside of the healthy range. They told me they ate most of their meals and snacks at home and visited sit-down restaurants from time to time. It turned out they were simply eating too much food. Their portion sizes were much larger than the recommended amounts. And often, their food wasn't prepared in a healthy manner.

One person talked about eating a large bowl of nuts as a snack on a regular basis. Hopefully he didn't eat as much as my husband, but I wouldn't be surprised if his large bowl contained close to, or even all, the total calories he needed in a day. While heart-healthy, nuts are high in calories and should only be eaten in small amounts.

I give my patients a "handy" guide for determining a serving size of nuts. Put the nuts in your hand. Close your hand comfortably. You aren't holding it shut with your other hand and nuts aren't falling out the sides. That's a serving size. About one serving size of fat (a category that nuts fall into) is good per meal.

Another attendee gasped when I held up a food model that showed the serving size of pasta. He said he ate at least *ten servings* at his meals. And there's always the delightful but calorie-deceitful avo-cado. A serving size is one-eighth of the avocado. Not a quarter, not a half, and most certainly not the whole thing. No one in that class, or in many of those I've taught, has said that they eat an appropriate portion size of avocado. By the way, one serving is 45 calories. So in the case of this particular class, they were eating too much of a lot of things. But they weren't doing it at fast food restaurants. They ate at home and at sit-down restaurants.

A study of more than 63,000 subjects reported in the *Journal of the American Medical Association* determined that portion sizes of desserts and hamburgers were larger when prepared and eaten at home rather than in a restaurant.

> If we're not careful, grocery shopping can be detrimental to our waistlines. Here are a couple of tips to help navigate around the store and avoid the plethora of less healthy, caloric food items:
>
> * Don't go to the grocery store hungry! When I've done this, I've on more than one occasion ended up placing empty wrappers of cookies/candies that I've already eaten on the conveyer belt at checkout.
> * Shop the perimeter of the store. The healthier items are there. But make an exception for the aisles that feature whole-grain items such as breads, cereals, rice and pastas.
> * Read food labels. It's important to know what we're buying. This enables us to make better choices.
> * Make a shopping list and stick to it!
> * Make a shopping list and stick to it!

Danger lurks at the grocery store as well. People eat two to three times more snack-type foods out of their shopping baskets while still in grocery stores than they do at fast food restaurants. And it matters what you place in that basket and bring home. We tend to eat what we buy. If we choose unhealthy items, we'll probably consume them. The same can be said of the more nutritious foods.

We can make not-so-good choices at the supermarket. But there are things that we can do to avoid this pitfall.

I always ask my patients if they would get in the car in Los Angeles and drive to New York without a road map and a basic driving plan. In this scenario, New York represents your long-term goal, such as "I want to lose 25 pounds." Sadly, we don't go to bed with that thought and wake up the next morning 25 pounds lighter. We need to map our route in order to reach the ultimate goal. One leg of the trip might be to eat three healthy balanced meals a day, another to consume appropriate portion sizes, and yet another to exercise for 60 minutes five days a week. Set your goals and plot the map to reach your long-term goal. The hospital where I work has an excellent tip for setting these short-term goals (or action plans). Make sure that on a scale of one to ten you have a confidence level of seven or above that you'll reach that goal. If you don't, rework the goal until you do. If we set a goal that we probably won't meet, we can get discouraged before we even begin. And when that happens, we may give up.

Be very specific in goal setting. We need to answer questions about what, where, when and how. A good action plan statement is: "I will walk on the treadmill for 60 minutes on Monday, Tuesday, Thursday, Friday and Saturday mornings." With this type of specificity, we can hold ourselves accountable and adjust the goals as needed.

The Road of Life

Lots of us are set in our ways and this definitely applies to our diets. Our lifestyles affect when, where, how and what we eat. There are always some who embrace change and actively seek to make healthier food choices. They're our role models, but not all of us are there yet. Therefore, we should make dietary changes to which we can comfortably adjust in the short term and maintain in the long term. We can then keep building on these changes to ultimately reach our goals.

It's easy to see that we just might be overdoing it, either in what and how much we're eating or in the action plans we set for ourselves. But rest assured, small changes can add up to big results. The first step is awareness. So let's take that path.

TEN

Setting the Table Straight

"We cannot deny that people are eating more and getting bigger, but that does not prove that fast food franchises are the culprit."

—Todd G. Buchholz, author of *Burgers, Fries and Lawyers: The Beef Behind Obesity Laws*

My husband and I love to eat out. Breakfast, lunch and dinner, you name it, we're there. And we're equal opportunity consumers. Fine dining establishments, middle-of-the-road sit-down restaurants, fast food, and sometimes even buffets have seen us cross their thresholds. I know what to look for and usually make healthy choices. It's not uncommon for me to ask for ingredients to be removed or added, or for the method of food preparation to be changed. For a good portion of my adult life, friends and family have likened me to Meg Ryan's fastidious character from the movie *When Harry Met Sally.* Like her, I'm usually very particular about what I eat. Many a waitperson has been at the receiving end of my sometimes long-winded orders. For a long time I was convinced I was eating very well at all the establishments. So, I was more than a little surprised when my weight started to creep up. And as a dietitian, I'm not alone. Kelly Brownell, director of the Rudd Center for Food Policy and Obesity at Yale points out that "even dietitians grossly underestimate the number of calories in dishes served at restaurants." He's right. And I was one of them.

Bring on the Data

My occasional underestimation of restaurant meal calories ended on July 1, 2009, when even dietitians got a wake-up call. On this date a new California law, SB 1420, began requiring restaurants with 20 or more locations to provide nutrition information on their menu offerings, including calories, grams of saturated fat, milligrams of sodium and grams of carbohydrate. Restaurants had to provide this information in one of the following ways:

- On a brochure or pamphlet on the table
- As an insert to the menu
- On the menu itself, adjacent to each standard item
- In an index of the menu, separate from the standard item listings
- On a table tent placed on the table

In addition, customers needed to be made aware that a brochure with nutrition information was available at the drive-thru window upon request. Effective January 2011, calorie information had to be posted next to each standard item on the menu board. Restaurants with table service had to provide calorie information next to each standard item on the menu. But, they are still required to also minimally provide information on total carbohydrate, total sodium and total saturated fat. Affected restaurants that don't have this information at the table are required to provide it upon request. I always ask, but I'm unhappy to say that I don't always get it. Kudos, though, to California Pizza Kitchen, which provides all the information in a take-home format. Sharing nutrition data is not specific to the United States. Fast food restaurants in Britain plan on embarking on voluntary menu labeling.

Unfortunately, some businesses aren't covered under the law, including grocery stores, convenience stores, farmers' markets and school cafeterias. So, there's work to be done.

But any information is better than none. It helps us make healthier decisions. It can be astonishing to see the nutrition facts for a lot of these restaurant meals, and not because the news is good.

McDonald's has some great nutrition features on its website (mcdonalds.com/). One is the "Bag a McMeal" section, where you can input items and calculate nutrition information for the entire meal. The "Simple Steps" section offers data on diabetic-friendly meals, including carbohydrate exchanges, lower sodium meals and cutting calories. The "Meal Comparison" section looks at how the Happy Meal stacks up to home-cooked meals. You might be surprised by the lower-calorie choice:

McDonald's Happy Meal	Ham Sandwich Meal
Chicken McNuggets (4 piece)	2 slices of bread
1% Low Fat Milk Jug	2 oz. of ham
Apple Slices	1 tsp. mayonnaise
Kids Fries	1 oz. potato chips
Fruit punch (8 fl. oz.)	
Cal 410	Cal 540
Fat 19 g	Fat 2 g

While lower in calories than the home-cooked example, the Happy Meal is higher in fat but it can have lower fat if you order only Apple Slices and no fries. I also don't like fried foods in general. So look for less high-fat items. The method of food preparation does matter.

California wasn't the only state to enact menu labeling legislation. Massachusetts, Maine, Oregon, Washington State, and Philadelphia have also passed similar laws. So did metro Nashville (Tennessee); New York City; Westchester, Albany, Ulster, and Suffolk counties in New York; King County (Seattle); and Multnomah County (Portland), among others.

As part of the 2010 health care reform legislation, a national standard for posting nutrition information will be established, with the FDA taking the lead in ironing out the details. Calorie labeling would be required on the menu boards and drive-thru displays of restaurants with 20 or more locations, as well as on vending machines. Additional nutrition information would have to be available upon request. This is all great.

But the reality is that some restaurants aren't in favor of this sharing of nutrition information. A high profile battle brewed in Manhattan between Hillstone Restaurant Group, the parent company of Houston's (a conventional sit-down restaurant chain), and the New York City Board of Health. At the time, Houston's had two locations in Manhattan. They changed the names of these restaurants to Hillstone in an apparent attempt to avoid having to comply with the new legislation. Hillstone refused to provide calorie content and other nutrition information on their menu. They said this was because the menu items at the two restaurants had different ingredients. Hillstone Restaurant Group was fined for their noncompliance but ultimately won the battle because of their name and menu changes.

In 2008, the New York City Board of Health faced more opposition. Dr. David B. Allison, president of the Obesity Society, wrote an affidavit supporting a lawsuit filed by the New York Restaurant Association against the menu labeling act. Dr. Allison stated that restaurant customers may not decrease their calorie intake with the posting of the nutrition information but in fact may *increase* it. He claimed that "by adding to the forbidden-fruit allure of high-calorie foods or by sending patrons away hungry enough that they will later gorge themselves even more," the strategy may backfire. The Obesity Society formally opposed Dr. Allison's statement.

And then there are the portion sizes. As I've said, they can be a major contributor to an expanding waistband. Often at sit-down restaurants, it's "one size fits all" meals, and the size is extra- large. For this reason, I usually only eat half of what's served me and take the rest home. But even though I do a lot of the right things, I found out when the California nutrition information laws went into effect that it often wasn't enough. One major point became clear: When comparing the calories, fat and sodium found in conventional sit-down restaurant menu items to those at fast food restaurants, the fast food offerings were often the healthier choice.

I'm ecstatic that most of my favorite restaurants must provide nutrition information on their menu offerings. And if you don't find everything that you want to know at the restaurants themselves, most of their websites have additional information. I look at this first, and when I find something that has a reasonable amount of calories and fat, I look at the item description and often modify its content through my order.

As you might guess, I spend a lot of time reading restaurant nutrition guides. They are fascinating to me. Here's a game I play with myself: I zoom in on the most caloric entrée on the menu just to see what all it contains. My jaw drops every time. Unfortunately, it's not just the most caloric item on the menu that can be problematic. The majority of sit-down restaurant menu choices can be a challenge. The food that I see being eaten as I walk to and from my table makes me want to stand up at the front of the restaurant and yell, "Time out!" But I rightfully resist. It's tough for me to see people in these establishments who are often eating more calories in one meal than they need *in an entire day*. It's not fast food, so it is better for them, right? Wrong.

There are far too many examples of excessive calories, fat and sodium at all the various restaurants for me to name. But I will mention a few. At Chili's, for example, if we order the Crispy Chicken

Crisper Tacos with rice and black beans and eat the whole plate, we would consume approximately 1,990 calories, 104 g fat, and 5,790 mg of sodium. Again I must repeat myself, but this is more calories and fat than many people should eat in an entire day, and (I hope you're sitting down) close to *three days'* worth of sodium intake. Even eating only half of the plate would provide many women with well over 50 percent of the recommended calorie intake for a day.

In the western United States, there's a restaurant chain called Claim Jumper that's known for its huge portions and admittedly very tasty food. For those who don't have this restaurant in your area, there's probably something similar near you. Just think of a local restaurant with very large plates piled high with food. If we dine at Claim Jumper and are in the mood for pasta, we might choose the Black Tie Chicken Pasta. If we eat the whole thing, we'll consume approximately 3,773 calories, 134 g of saturated fat and 4,638 mg of sodium. Even eating a half order can cost us an entire day's worth of calories. That half portion contains 2,035 calories, 71 g of saturated fat and 2,541 mg of sodium.

Even many of the restaurant's entrée salads (as is true of so many conventional sit-down restaurants) have far too many calories. We're not eating light by ordering the *small* citrus chicken salad. It has 1,497 calories, 21 g of saturated fat and 877 mg of sodium.

Claim Jumper is also one of many sit-down chains that serve mega-sized burgers. It even calls one the Widow Maker Burger, which weighs in at a total of 1,492 calories, 29 g of saturated fat and 2,648 mg of sodium. The name alone should make us wary, but the calorie, fat and sodium content should make us shudder. But I don't need to just pick on Claim Jumper. There are many sit-down restaurants that offer the oversized hamburger. One is Cheesecake Factory, which has a Tons of Fun Burger that packs on approximately 1,400 calories and 2030 mg of sodium. If we eat too many of those, it's likely we'll be having a lot less fun in general.

In Arizona, Las Vegas and Dallas, there's a restaurant called Heart Attack Grill that serves up unhealthy fare, with a focus on hamburgers. Their menu includes the Quadruple Bypass Burger (8,000 calories); Flatliner Fries, deep-fried in lard; and butterfat milkshakes. The waitresses wear nurse uniforms and anyone who weighs 350 pounds or more gets to eat for free. In March 2011, Heart Attack Grill lost its 29-year-old spokesperson, Blair River, when he died after suffering a bout of pneumonia. He weighed 575 pounds. In early 2012, a male patron suffered an apparent heart attack at the restaurant while eating the 6,000-calorie Triple Bypass Burger. More recently, a woman eating at the Las Vegas location also had an apparent heart attack. She had chosen a smaller but still too-large menu choice, the Double Bypass Burger. The Heart Attack Grill's slogan is: "A Burger to Die For." It appears that some of the restaurant's customers may be on their way to doing exactly that.

The calorie and fat composition of meals at sit-down restaurants can be so bad that one study found that "a proliferation of full-service restaurants would raise obesity levels more than a proliferation of fast food establishments."

A USDA survey found that pasta portions eaten by Americans were 333 percent larger and muffin sizes were 480 percent bigger than recommended portions. These are not typically items found at fast food restaurants, although the beloved and less criticized coffee houses certainly sell a lot of massive muffins. So do supermarkets and warehouse stores. These statistics led Todd G. Buchholz, author of *Burgers, Fries and Lawyers*, to write, "If we are turning into a jumbo people, we are a jumbo people everywhere we eat…"

In 2012, *Consumer Reports* surveyed 47,565 people who consumed 110,517 meals at 102 sit-down restaurant chains. Of those earning the highest marks in the seven categories analyzed, Biaggi's Ristorante Italiano was admired for "focusing on big portions."

Starbucks muffins are also a good example of big portions. Their Blueberry Scone has 460 calories and 22 grams of fat. The Banana Nut Loaf has 490 calories and 19 grams of fat. The Cranberry Orange Scone has 490 calories and 18 grams of fat.

Let's Dish

While not all restaurants are required to post nutrition information, the good news is we can find it through a variety of means. There are many calorie tracking books out there, including *The Calorie King Calorie, Fat & Carbohydrate Counter*, which is updated annually. Other books I like are the aforementioned *Eat This Not That!* series, Bob Greene's *The Get with the Program Guide to Fast Food & Family Restaurants*, and Hope S. Warshaw's *Guide to Healthy Restaurant Eating* and *Guide to Healthy Fast-Food Eating* (yes, healthy), which she wrote for the American Diabetes Association.

Greene is a certified personal trainer and exercise physiologist who specializes in weight loss, metabolism and fitness. He's Oprah Winfrey's personal trainer and was a frequent guest on her show. He's a contributing writer and editor for *O, The Oprah Magazine* and is a bestselling author of several healthy eating and lifestyle books, two of which were co-authored by Winfrey. He also worked as a consultant for McDonald's and its healthy lifestyles public awareness campaign. With McDonald's, Greene began the McDonald's Go Active! American Challenge in May 2004. As part of the program, he walked and bicycled over 3,000 miles in 36 days, visiting McDonald's restaurants along the way.

Greene developed the *Step With It!* fitness booklet for the McDonald's Go Active! Happy Meal for adults. It included a Premium Salad, pedometer, the *Step With It!* booklet and bottled water or a fountain drink. It was estimated that ten to 15 million pedometers and fitness books were given out to customers and organizations across the United States. "McDonald's and I are working together to continue educating people about leading balanced, active lifestyles—realistically and for the long term," says Greene. "As a leader in the food industry, McDonald's has a unique opportunity to reach out to people on so many levels. Together we are committed to helping people make better choices through food and energy balance." "Realistically," "long-term," "better choices"—these are words that I use every day with patients.

Besides books, there are other sources that can sometimes provide the less-accessible nutrition information for sit-down restaurants. Sites like **nutritiondata.com, calorieking.com,** and **caloriecount.com** cover many different restaurants. A good way to keep a food diary and track calories is **myfitnesspal.com.** Unfortunately, not all of the data for conventional sit-down restaurants can be found on these websites either. When Warshaw wrote in one of her books, "Honesty is their policy. Full disclosure of nutrition information is there for the asking," she was not speaking about the sit-down restaurants. She was referring to fast food establishments.

Around the time that menu labeling began in California, my husband and I had dinner at the Italian restaurant chain Romano's Macaroni Grill. When we received our food, the portion sizes were smaller than normal. I thought this was a positive, not a negative, as the serving size of my entrée seemed more appropriate for a single portion. While we were eating, I heard a waitress explaining that the portion sizes had indeed gotten smaller when the chain began printing nutrition information on its menus.

I asked Larry Nedwed, senior brand manager for Macaroni Grill, if what the waitress said was indeed the case. He maintained it wasn't. "These changes were part of a new direction to offer consumers a menu of Italian food that is amongst other things better for you… not as a response to the state's menu labeling laws," he said. Either way, I applaud the move.

If You Use It, You May Lose It

At least we're moving in the right direction. I'm happy to report that even my food-loving husband has taken notice and has started to use the provided nutrition facts (every now and then), admittedly after much prompting from his caring wife. When he found out that his favorite hamburger (the Kilauea) at Islands Bar & Grill had 1,600 calories, 36 g of saturated fat and 2,320 mg of sodium, not including sides, he made a change. While he used to eat the whole burger, he now eats half of it and takes the rest home. But more and more, he'll order an entirely different menu item, one that's much lower in calories, fat and sodium. This is what we all should do the majority of the time. But do we?

The city of New York predicts that in the next several years, menu labeling will result in 150,000 fewer New Yorkers becoming obese and 30,000 fewer developing diabetes. And because studies have shown that people aren't good at estimating the calorie content of the food they eat at restaurants, it stands to reason that providing this information would be helpful. But once we know, do we change?

One study found that after the menu labeling law was instituted in New York, consumers ordered meals that had a mean of 846 calories. Prior to the law, the mean calories consumed were 825. While this may not seem like a huge difference, it's still more calories consumed and that's not the direction we'd expect.

The real question is, how do we choose what we eat in restaurants? Research shows that overall, taste is the main reason given for choosing the entrée, whether there was nutrition information or not. (After taste, people's priorities are price and healthfulness, in that order). A study published by the National Bureau of Economic Research found that labeling helped decrease obesity, but only in white, non-Hispanic women. There was no significant impact for black and Hispanic women, as well as men in all ethnic groups. This is definitely concerning.

I discuss reading the nutrition facts in menus and on packaged food labels in just about every class I teach. Many of my patients are very proactive and review the information provided to them. But a significant number don't notice or look at the materials at all, even if they know they're there for them to see. This is probably indicative of the general population. Hopefully, we'll continue to find ways to get more of us to use the provided information and to make healthy changes in our lives. We can't reasonably expect massive changes overnight, but at least in the city of New York there are some encouraging signs that these efforts are working. A 2008 study by Technomics focusing on the effectiveness of menu labeling in New York City garnered some positive results:

- 84 percent of restaurant customers used the nutrition information provided to them.
- 84 percent were surprised by the calorie content of foods, finding them to be higher than expected.
- 75 percent believed the nutrition information affected their ordering.

I'd like to know where the biggest surprise in calorie content came from. I suspect it was from the conventional sit-down restaurants, particularly after seeing all the nutrition facts on menus here in California. Believe me, I've practically fainted at least a hundred times. And many of my patients and clients have as well. Perhaps even a few tears have been shed.

It's important to note that calorie counts aren't always accurate. I'm asked about this all the time. Many doubt what they read, and sometimes we should be skeptical. A recent Tufts University study found that ten frozen meals bought from grocery stores had, on average, 8 percent more calories than their nutrition labels said. For example, Lean Cuisine's shrimp and angel hair pasta had 319 calories, not the 220 calories specified on the label.

Of the 29 sit-down and fast food restaurants studied, actual calories averaged 18 percent higher than stated. Some of these included Denny's dry toast with 283 calories, not the 92 listed. And, Denny's grits had 258 calories, not the reported 80. P.F. Chang's large Sichuan-style asparagus had more than double the number of calories listed in the menu. Fast food restaurants were not immune to miscalculations either. McDonald's McChicken sandwich had 3 percent more calories than the indicated 360, and Wendy's Ultimate Chicken Grill had 9 percent more than the listed 320. A pat on the back to Domino's and its thin crust cheese pizza, which was found to have 141 calories, not the stated 180. Also, Denny's overreported by 6 percent the number of calories in its dry English muffin.

So be careful and take these numbers with a grain of salt. Figuratively, not literally, please. Also, be particularly mindful of sit-down restaurants' nutritional information, because as already mentioned, the calories and other nutrition information often don't include what comes on the entire plate. In the Tufts study, five of the restaurants' side dishes added an average of 471 additional calories to the calories listed for the entrée.

The Food and Drug Administration (FDA) allows a 20 percent margin of error for the calorie count of packaged foods.

Size Wise

One of the big differences between sit-down restaurants and fast food fare is the portion size. But where does the real "supersizing" take place? Clearly, if we go to a fast food restaurant and order any sandwich with double, triple or quadruple in its name, and/or large fries, and/or a large regular soda, we've "supersized." We've simply made our meal too large and too calorie- and fat-laden.

If we go to a fast food restaurant and order a combo meal, in some cases we have the choice of ordering bigger versions of items like the fries and the drinks. The key word here is *choice*. No one makes us order the larger portions. We're not threatened, harassed or cajoled in any way. It's offered to us, and if we decline, there are no repercussions. The ball is in our court. Conversely, no one stops us if we order too much at a fast food restaurant. But why would they? And what would we think if they did? I've often seen many people order too much food for a single meal, but I don't walk up to them and lecture them on their choice. It wouldn't be accepted or appropriate.

For the most part, just about everything at a fast food restaurant can be à la carte. We're able to customize our own quantity. This includes soda (which hopefully is diet). We can choose a smaller-size cup if we want, and we should. And if we order at the drive-thru, we won't be tempted by the free refills.

In 2010, the ABC News hidden camera television show *What Would You Do?* orchestrated public displays in which wait staff at a restaurant discouraged obese actors, posing as patrons, from ordering calorie-laden food. Unsuspecting diners who overheard the exchanges primarily expressed outrage at the actions of the wait staff and consoled the obese actor, who they thought was just a restaurant diner like themselves. Most of us would respond that way, and rightfully so. We don't want restaurant workers to tell us what we should and shouldn't eat.

We don't get as many à la carte options at sit-down restaurants, and what we get is often too large. And what do we do when we get our plate? We eat a lot (if not all) of it. In fact, studies have found that when served larger portions, people will "step up to the plate." Specifically, one study revealed that when diners were presented with a larger portion of a popular pasta dish, they consumed much more of it. This is a huge problem for our bellies, hips and thighs.

Did You Save Room for Dessert?

The individual portion sizes at sit-down restaurants aren't the only thing that leads us to overeat. Think a moment about how we get our food at these types of restaurants. Do we order at a menu board? No. Someone comes to our table to take our order. And while we call them wait staff, make no mistake about it, they're salespeople.

In *Chew On This*, Eric Schlosser and Charles Wilson discuss the carhops at drive-in restaurants and the part they played in the McDonald brothers' decision to open a drive-in restaurant of their own: "[The carhops] earned money from tips and received a small share of the money their customers spent. The more food and drinks a customer ordered, the more money a carhop earned. As a result, carhops tended to be very nice to their customers and encouraged them to eat and drink a lot." I don't know about you, but that sounds like most every waitperson who comes to my table at a sit-down restaurant. And who can blame them? After all, their tip is almost always based on the total amount of food and drinks purchased. If I were them, I'd do the same exact thing. It's a different experience from the fast food counterperson, who might ask us once if we want a large version of a menu item. At a sit-down restaurant, however, we're asked throughout the meal if we want to order additional items or get refills. Then at the end of our meal, the waitperson often brings over a beautifully decorated dessert tray to showcase the delicious delights that are ours just for the asking. Many of us take them up on the offer.

So what's the result? Often at these sit-down restaurants, we don't just eat the entrée. We bookend the meal with an appetizer and a dessert. For those who drink sugary sodas and juice with their food, many sit-down restaurants continually refill their glasses, adding another whopping number of calories to the meal. Alcoholic beverages add calories as well. And there is that pesky bread/tortilla-filled basket that appears on the table, often before we even order, and is refilled throughout the meal. Remember, a little goes a long way. Take a look...

Bread Item	Approximate Calories
Cheesecake Factory Brown Bread - 2 slices	88
Macaroni Grill Peasant Bread - ¼ piece	120
Olive Garden Breadstick - 1	150
Red Lobster Cheddar Bay Biscuit - 1	140

It's not impossible for someone to go to a sit-down restaurant and eat two, three, or even four days' worth of calories in one sitting. And I'm not talking about a buffet. So it's absolutely critical that we don't ignore these restaurants as a significant contributor to our expanding waistlines and potential health problems.

It's Good for You...Or Is It?

Mention should be made of the restaurants we consider "healthy." Do we actually eat better at them? Research from Cornell University suggests we don't. "We found that when people go to restaurants claiming to be healthy, such as Subway, they choose additional side items containing up to 131 percent more calories than when they go to restaurants like McDonald's that don't make that claim," says study co-author Brian Wansink, professor of marketing and applied economics and director of the Cornell Food and Brand Lab. The study also found that when eating at so-called "healthy restaurants," diners typically underestimated their calorie intake by 35 percent.

I find this to be especially true at the salad buffet restaurants. Okay, just the word "buffet" says it all, but these restaurants exist, and it's certainly possible to eat appropriate amounts of food at them. No one takes our hand, puts a serving spoon in it, and makes us fill our plates to overflowing. But so many of us behave as if they do. If you're not familiar with this dining concept, it features a long salad bar that contains many types of vegetables, as well as an assortment of creamy/mayonnaise-based salads, cheese, croutons, olives, and the like. At the end of the line, the diner pays before moving on to other stations for pasta, pizza, muffins, soups, drinks and desserts. One price typically covers all you can eat.

I absolutely adore these soup and salad bar restaurants and often frequent one near where I live. When my husband and I go, I start at the beginning of the line and pick my favorite lettuce and a varied selection of fresh vegetables. I don't choose any of the creamy/mayonnaise-based salads, and I only put about a tablespoon of fat-free dressing on my plate. Further, I don't put cheese, croutons, wontons, or anything of that nature on my very healthy concoction. When we get to the point of payment, I have a very colorful plate of low-calorie, low-fat, nutritious food. My husband's tray is a different matter. Invariably, the plate on it is *empty*. Not even a leaf of lettuce graces it. He's not at the restaurant for that. His pleasure lies beyond.

> While a serving size of regular salad dressing is one tablespoon and reduced calorie/nonfat dressing is two tablespoons, I never see a tablespoon-size serving utensil provided. It's always a ladle. And through my measurement enterprise, I've learned these ladles hold about three tablespoons. Even if we pour only one ladle of dressing on our salads, we've already poured too much. Any many of us don't stop at one.

By the time we get to our table, in addition to my salad, I've added a small baked potato with approximately one-quarter cup of reduced fat cottage cheese and one small reduced-fat fruit muffin. My husband, on the other hand, arrives at the table with nothing but what I call "brown food": pizza, pasta, full-fat muffins and chili. And when I get up for my healthy dessert, fruit, he goes back for his second round of the brown food. He typically doesn't get his dessert until his third trip. And it's never a piece of fruit. In a restaurant packed with nutritious food, he's zeroed in on some of the less healthy choices. Believe me, I continue to work on him. But we have to make our own choices. No one can do it for us.

The amount of food we heap on our plates at soup and salad buffets (or any type of buffet, for that matter) can be absolutely astonishing. Many do start with vegetables, but by the time we reach the cash register, we've covered these vegetables with high-fat, high-calorie cheese, croutons and fat-laden concoctions such as macaroni and potato salads. We then place one, two, sometimes even three ladles of high-fat dressing over the top of this massive pile. We know that even one ladle is too much. But we've only just begun. We then move on to the hot section and load up on pasta, pizza and bread. Later we go back for dessert. It's easy to see salad isn't always the low-calorie dish we think it is. Ingredients matter.

So, given the sheer size of the portions served at many conventional sit-down restaurants, their often less healthy methods of food preparation, and the amounts and types of food we load on our plates at buffets, it can be difficult to build a healthy meal. Surprisingly to some, we can find a similar menu item at a fast food restaurant with better nutrition content. Unfortunately, both fast food and sit-down restaurants flunk when it comes to sodium content.

For those not on a sodium-restricted diet, it's recommended that we consume no more than 1,500 mg of sodium per day. To put this in perspective, one teaspoon of salt has about 2,325 mg. One large dill pickle has about 1,430. Canned goods that aren't of the "no salt added" variety, frozen meals, cured meats and certain condiments and sauces are just a few of the high-sodium foods we eat every day. Not surprisingly, the average American consumes about 3,400 mg of sodium a day.

In *Don't Eat This Book,* Spurlock again focused on fast food restaurants. He thinks their menu items shouldn't "even be called food." Instead, he sees them as a "highly efficient delivery system for fats, carbohydrates, sugars and other bad things." In some cases he's right and we should heed his warning. He rightfully points out that a big culprit is the french fry and says the typical American consumes approximately 30 pounds of fries each year. That's a huge quantity, to be sure.

A medium baked potato has about 164 calories. French fries made from that same potato, if deep fried, would contain about 578 calories.

Spurlock also says children drink double the amount of sugary sodas than they did 25 years ago. That's a 135 percent increase in the intake of soft drinks between 1977 and 2001. Not good.

The USDA reported that the average person in the U.S. eats 30 pounds more sugar annually than we did 30 years ago. We also consume more meat (20 pounds), more cheese (14 pounds), more white flour (35 pounds), and more fat (12 pounds).

Spurlock and others focus on fast food. But we need to look at *all* restaurants and other areas where we dine to get a true sense of this overindulgence of food. My husband drinks a two-liter bottle of Mountain Dew at home every day. At least it's the diet variety, but it's still too much. Many sit-down restaurants continually refill our sodas, typically without us even having to ask. More and more when I'm at a sit-down restaurant, I'm asked if I'd like a refill to-go beverage when I get my check. Fast food restaurants often place their soda fountains in the seating area to facilitate refills.

With regard to french fries, it's true you can get a large order of fries at fast food restaurants. That's too much, and french fries shouldn't be ordered most of the time. But sit- down restaurants can be worse. More than a few serve unlimited french fries. It's bottomless.

The following table illustrates the nutrition content of similar menu items at a variety of fast food and sit-down restaurants.

FAST FOOD VINDICATION

Sit-Down Restaurant	Menu Item	Cal	Fat (g)	Sodium (mg)	Fast Food Restaurant	Menu Item	Cal	Fat (g)	Sodium (mg)
Bob Evans	Grilled Chicken (1 piece—plain)	214	9	544	Kentucky Fried Chicken	Grilled Chicken Breast	180	4	n/a
						Chicken Breast—no skin or breading	140	2	n/a
Chili's	Crispy Chicken Crisper Tacos (2—no sides)	1,190	74	3,130	Taco Bell	Crunchy Taco Supreme (2)	400	24	700
	Chicken Tacos (2)	600	29	2,110		Fresco Crunch Taco (2)	300	14	700
	Quesadilla Explosion Salad	1,270	76	2,650		Chipotle Steak Fully Loaded Taco Salad	950	59	1,760
	Southern Smokehouse Bacon Big Mouth Burger (no sides)	1,630	108	4,170	Carl's Jr	Double Western Bacon Cheeseburger	960	52	1,750

Sit-Down Restaurant	Menu Item	Cal	Fat (g)	Sodium (mg)
	Bacon Burger (no sides)	1,090	69	1,800
	Oldtimer (no sides)	820	44	1,310
Coco's	Original Burger (no sides)	760	12 Sat Fat	1,690
	Bacon Cheddar Burger (no sides)	970	20 Sat Fat	2,100
	Classic Burger (no sides)	694	35	785
Friday's	Bacon Cheeseburger (no sides)	1,360	n/a	n/a
	Friday's Cheeseburger	1,310	n/a	n/a

Fast Food Restaurant	Menu Item	Cal	Fat (g)	Sodium (mg)
	Western Bacon Cheeseburger	710	33	1,410
	Low Carb Six Dollar Burger	490	37 / 6	1,290
Burger King	Hamburger	290	Sat Fat 14	560
	Whopper with Cheese	610	Sat Fat	1,310
	Single with everything	430	20	870
Jack in the Box	Jumbo Jack	600	35	940
Jack in the Box	Ultimate Cheeseburger	1,010	71	1,580

FAST FOOD VINDICATION

Sit-Down Restaurant	Menu Item	Cal	Fat (g)	Sodium (mg)
	All-American Grilled Chicken Sandwich (no sides)	730	n/a	n/a
Ruby Tuesday	Classic Burger	830	53	n/a
	Bacon Cheeseburger	1009	67	n/a
	Low Carb Chicken Caesar Salad	501	35	n/a

Fast Food Restaurant	Menu Item	Cal	Fat (g)	Sodium (mg)
	Jack's Spicy Chicken	620	31	1,100
McDonald's	Hamburger	250	9	520
	Quarter Pounder	410	19	730
	Big N' Tasty	460	24	720
	Big Mac	540	29	1,040
	Cheeseburger	300	12	750
	Grilled Chicken Caesar Salad (with dressing)	410	24	1,390
	Grilled Chicken Caesar salad (no dressing)	220	6	890

As you can see, often the listed fast food choices have less calories, fat and sodium than the sit-down counterparts. This illustrates that we need to be mindful of everywhere we eat. Fast food isn't always the worst choice. But it's not always the best choice either. Clearly, more than a few of the menu items listed weren't the healthiest choices.

So what do I recommend at a fast food restaurant? Single hamburgers, grilled chicken sandwiches, turkey burgers or veggie burgers (none with mayonnaise or cheese), salads with grilled chicken and low-fat/nonfat, low-calorie dressing), skinless chicken breasts, yogurt parfaits, baked potatoes, carrot sticks and apple slices, to name a few. The choices are numerous and growing as these establishments add healthier menu items. The following gives an example of some better choices we can make at a fast food restaurant.

Burger King
1 Tendergrill Chicken Sandwich, no mayo, 1 side Garden Salad without croutons and with 2 tbsp Fat Free Honey Mustard Dressing, 1 order Apple Fries
Nutrition Facts: Calories 510, Total Fat 7 g, Saturated Fat 1.5 g, Trans Fat 0 g, Percent Calories from Fat 12, Sodium 1,230 mg, Carbohydrate 77 g

1 Fire-Grilled Chicken Garden Salad with 2 tbsp Fat Free Honey Mustard Dressing, 1 Strawberry Apple Sauce
Nutrition Facts: Calories 437, Total Fat 14 g, Saturated Fat 6 g, Trans Fat 0 g, Percent Calories from Fat 29, Sodium 1,767 mg, Carbohydrate 53 g

KFC
1 Oven-Roasted Breast without skin or breading, 1 large Corn-on-the-Cob, 1 order Green Beans
Nutrition Facts: Calories 340, Total Fat 8 g, Saturated Fat 2 g, Trans Fat 0 g, Percent Calories from Fat 21, Sodium 990 mg, Carbohydrate 33 g

1 Honey Barbecue Sandwich, 1 Order Mashed Potatoes without gravy, 1 order Green Beans
Nutrition Facts: Calories 440, Total Fat 9 g, Saturated Fat 3 g, Trans Fat 0.5 g, Percent Calories from Fat 18.4, Sodium 1,361 mg, Carbohydrate 57 g

McDonald's
Egg McMuffin and 1 snack size Fruit 'n Yogurt Parfait without granola
Nutrition Facts: Calories 430, Total Fat 14 g, Saturated Fat 6 g, Trans Fat, 0 g, Percent calories from Fat 29, Sodium 875 mg, Carbohydrate 55 g

1 California Cobb Salad with Grilled Chicken and 2 tbsp (1/2 packet) Newman's Own Cobb Dressing, 1 Fruit 'n Yogurt Parfait without granola
Nutrition Facts: Calories 470, Total Fat 17 g, Saturated Fat 7 g, Trans Fat 0 g, Percent Calories from Fat 33, Sodium 1,615 mg, Carbohydrate 46 g

1 Regular Hamburger, Side Salad with 2 tbsp Newman's Own Low Fat Balsamic Vinaigrette, Vanilla Reduced Fat Ice Cream Cone
Nutrition Facts: Calories 460, Total Fat 15.5 g, Saturated Fat 5.5 g, Trans Fat 0.5 g, Percent Calories from Fat 30, Sodium 1,320 mg, Carbohydrate 63g

Taco Bell
2 Fresco Grilled Steak Soft Tacos, 1 order Pintos 'N Cheese
Nutrition Facts: Calories 490, Total Fat 15 g, Saturated Fat 6 g, Trans Fat 0 g, Percent Calories from Fat 28, Sodium 1,610 mg, Carbohydrate 60 g

1 Fresco Burrito Supreme (Chicken), 1 order Mexican Rice
Nutrition Facts: Calories 470, Total Fat 11.5 g, Saturated Fat 2.5 g, Trans Fat 0 g, Percent Calories from Fat 22, Sodium 1,800 mg, Carbohydrate 70 g

<u>Wendy's</u>

1 large Chili, 1 Side Salad with 2 tbsp (1/2 packet) Reduced Fat Creamy Ranch Dressing, 1 Mandarin Orange Cup

Nutrition Facts: Calories 445, Total Fat 13 g, Saturated Fat 4.25 g, Trans Fat 0.5 g, Percent Calories from Fat 26, Sodium 1,500 mg, Carbohydrate 58 g

1 Ultimate Chicken Grill Sandwich, 1 Kid's Meal Fries

Nutrition Facts: Calories 530, Total Fat 17 g, Saturated Fat 3 g, Trans Fat 0 g, Percent Calories from Fat 29, Sodium 1,130 g, Carbohydrate 64 g

The above recommendations cover a wide variety of tastes. So there's probably something for all of us in there. I even included items such as rice, pintos and cheese, small fries and reduced-fat ice cream in some of the meal combinations, so you can see that treats aren't completely off the table. But take a good hard look at the sodium content. It's too high across the board. This is definitely an area for improvement.

ELEVEN

There's No Place Like Home

"Chef Paul Prudhomme is a hero of mine, a man who sacrificed his life for that fine, buttery creamy cooking. I can at least do it for a year. But I don't think even Julia herself would suggest eating like this every day of the week is a healthy lifestyle."

—Julie Powell, author of *Julie and Julia: My Year of Cooking Dangerously*

Critics of the fast food industry often point to home-cooked meals as a better nutritional option, but is it really? Some might be surprised to learn that there are more calories and fat in many foods prepared and served at home. And with quite a few meals being eaten at home and other non-fast food venues, it becomes even more difficult to entirely blame fast food for the skyrocketing obesity rates.

> Psychiatrist Daniel Amen recently made a very keen observation, "Go to church...get donuts...bacon...sausage...hot dogs...ice cream. They have no idea they are sending people to heaven EARLY!" Church is certainly not fast food. Food items and dishes that often find themselves at potlucks are often items that we prepare at home and take with us where we go.

Not long ago, the #2 bestselling book on the *New York Times* nonfiction list was *Mastering the Art of French Cooking* by Julia Child, Louisette Bertholle and Simone Beck. The increased popularity of this over-40-year-old cookbook was due to the then-current movie, *Julie & Julia,* which chronicles the true story of Julie Powell, who cooked every recipe in the cookbook, while interweaving the tale of how Child created the book itself. We can only assume that because so many people were buying it, many tried cooking a recipe or two at home for their families and friends to enjoy. I'm sure the meals were very tasty, yet they probably weren't so healthy. But the casual reader wouldn't know that at a glance. There's no nutrition information for the recipes anywhere in the book.

French cuisine is delicious. And Julia Child helped introduce it to millions of households in America and around the world. But a cookbook written over 40 years ago probably didn't keep health and nutrition top of mind. Fat and calories run rampant in Child's recipes. You'll find lots of both in the Hollandaise sauce. In *Mastering the Art of French Cooking*, the ingredients for three-quarters of a cup of Hollandaise sauce are:

3 egg yolks
¼ tsp salt

pinch of pepper
1 to 2 tbsp lemon juice
4 ounces or 1 stick of butter

This concoction contains approximately 978 calories and 105 grams of fat. No, I'm not kidding. One fat gram equals nine calories (compared to one gram of protein or carbohydrate, which are four calories). With 105 grams of total fat, the Hollandaise sauce in question has 945 calories from fat.

And the above ingredients are the amounts needed for making the sauce in the blender. If a blender isn't used, the recipe would call for eight to nine ounces of butter. This would add approximately 812 more calories and 92 grams of fat. This is just the sauce.

Flipping through Child's cookbook, many of the recipes have ingredients like heavy whipping cream, whole milk, whole eggs and egg yolks, butter, oil, etc. And on top of these calorie-laden recipes, Americans eating this fare are probably consuming far more than would the French, because the U.S. idea of portion sizes is larger than the Gallic, and probably more than what Child intended. In fact, Julie Powell, the author of *Julie & Julia: My Year of Cooking Dangerously*, suffered the consequences. She gained 20 pounds over her yearlong project. Some of this was brought on by the 60 to 70 pounds of butter she used in the recipes throughout the year.

My husband and I recently took a trip to Paris, where we had a wonderful time. But, on our first night there, my "better half" had a bit of a rude awakening while dining out in a local restaurant. He placed his order and upon receipt of his meal, he took one look at it, frowned and proclaimed, "I have been gypped! They didn't give me the right amount of food!" I took a look at his plate and saw that they had not cut his portion size to an unreasonable amount. They had given him what was appropriate, but he did not think so, because our portion sizes are so exaggerated in the United States.

FAST FOOD VINDICATION

Some might say a 40-year-old cookbook, even one that was a recent bestseller, isn't a good representation of how we eat today or how contemporary cookbooks are written. If you think that, you're mistaken. There are current cookbooks that lack nutrition information and feature ingredients and quantities that are less than healthy. And I'm sorry to report that I'm not talking about only a few. There are many. Why not open the cookbooks you have at home and see if they make the grade?

To make matters worse, a recent study directed by Cornell University marketing professor Brian Wansink found many cookbooks have "supersized" their recipes. Calories have increased by almost 40 percent a serving over the past 70 years for almost every classic recipe reviewed in a variety of cookbooks. That's about 77 extra calories.

The researchers looked closely at the *Joy of Cooking*, which was first published in the 1930s and has been updated over the years—most recently in 2006. Of 18 recipes found in all seven editions, researchers found an average 17-calorie increase per serving in the latest edition. The only recipe that didn't change was the chili con carne. Part of the reason for the increase in calories was the change in portion sizes. *They got bigger.* One of the dishes the researchers looked at was the Chicken Gumbo. In the first edition, the recipe made 14 servings with 228 calories per serving. In the 2006 edition, the recipe makes only 10 portions with 576 calories each. When asked about this "calorie creep," the editor of *Joy of Cooking* explained that the revisions follow industry standards and reflect a fundamental change in the way Americans produce and consume food. Unfortunately she's right.

Like cookbooks, some of the many cooking magazines on the market are better than others as far as providing healthy recipes with corresponding nutrition information. On a recent trip to the bookstore, I picked up a variety of them. All of the healthy-eating periodicals contained nutrition information. So when we cook these recipes, we know what we're eating in the form of calories, fat, etc. But those magazines that feature heavier, less-healthy dishes often neglect to clue us in on just how many calories and fat we're actually eating. Then there are some, like *Food Network Magazine,* that only provide nutrition information for some of their recipes. Why not all of them? Others such as *Bon Appetite* don't provide any. With recipes like Layered Brownies with White-Chocolate Caramel and Cacao Nib Gelato, one can perhaps see why. I'm betting they're yummy but probably not so good on the tummy.

Another popular magazine, *Paula Deen's Best Dishes*, from celebrity chef Paula Deen, has no nutrition information either and a fair amount of calorie- and fat-laden recipes. In her foreword from one issue, she writes, "In this issue, I'm going to share with you some of the best hearty recipes from my magazine. Treat it as a prized cookbook to pull out when you're looking for the perfect comfort dish to make for your family on a cool night, or when you're in a hurry and want something simple and quick but full of flavor. I hope it's a book you'll come back to time and time again for favorite meals and ideas. May my treasured recipes warm your heart and home for many meals to come." With ingredients like whole milk, heavy whipping cream, butter, creamy soups, bacon, ham, cheese (not reduced fat or no-fat) and sour cream (not reduced fat or no-fat), some of her recipes may do more than *warm* your heart.

Let's take a look at her Crunchy Nacho Cheese Chicken Casserole. It serves eight to ten people and has among other ingredients:

2 tablespoons of butter
16 ounces of regular sour cream
two 10.75-ounce cans of cream of chicken soup (not a light version)
one 13-ounce bag of nacho cheese-flavored tortilla chips
1 cup of shredded Monterey Jack cheese (the full-fat version)
1 cup of shredded regular Cheddar cheese

As we can see, this recipe and others like it, while undoubtedly delicious, shouldn't be enjoyed every day. While interviewing Deen on *The View* about a children's cookbook she'd written, broadcast legend Barbara Walters expressed some concern about the nutritional content of the recipes. Deen gave the appropriate response, saying that some of her recipes should be viewed as treats or foods for special occasions. She's right. Remember, moderation is the key.

> Encouraging a child to "clean your plate or you won't get dessert" can backfire on parents. Studies have shown by the time children reach the age of five, they've learned to clean their plate. Younger kids don't seem to have yet picked up on that behavior. They often tend to stop eating when they're satisfied.

Deen recently announced she has type 2 diabetes. She acknowledged that it took her some time to make appropriate lifestyle changes, but she seems to be doing so now. She's lost weight by reducing the calories and fat in the foods she eats. Her son Bobby now has his own cooking show that takes Deen's recipes and lightens them up, making them more healthy. Recently a piece on the *Today* show discussed how her diagnosis would affect her brand. It remains to be seen.

> Just because a recipe calls for less healthy ingredients doesn't mean we have to prepare the dish that way. Look for substitutions such as:
>
> * Nonfat or 1% milk instead of whole or 2% milk
> * Low-fat or nonfat cheeses for regular cheese
> * Egg whites or egg substitutes instead of whole eggs
> * Unsaturated oils (olive, peanut, canola) over coconut, palm and palm kernel oils
> *Cut the oil content in half—or better yet, replace it entirely – with spray-on butter/oil that's lightly sprayed on the pan/dish
> * Nonfat yogurt or reduced-calorie mayonnaise instead of regular mayonnaise
> * Lean ground turkey or ground beef over ground chuck

There's No Place Like Home

Cornell University's Wansink sums it up: "There's so much attention that's been given to away-from-home eating and so much attention that's been focused on restaurants and the packaged food industry, it makes me wonder whether it's actually deflecting attention from the one place where we can make the most immediate change." He's right. I challenge you to take a look at your favorite recipes. Do they have calorie-and fat-laden ingredients? Do they contain nutrition information? Are you eating them in the recommended serving sizes? Do you know how much you're actually consuming in your home-cooked meals?

It's something to chew on…

Packaged/Processed Foods

Not too long ago my mother called to let me know she'd just been diagnosed with prediabetes, which exists when a person has abnormally high blood glucose readings, but not at levels elevated enough to be diagnosed with diabetes. My co-workers and I call prediabetes "diet-controlled diabetes." People with prediabetes often go on to develop diabetes within a number of years, so it's essential that preventative efforts begin immediately.

My mother was naturally upset by her diagnosis but was very willing to do what was needed to help keep her blood sugar under control. She wanted my help. I asked her what she typically ate in one day, a lot of which I already knew. She definitely had a sweet tooth and loved those 100-calorie-pack cookies. These aren't too bad if we eat just one package, but she was known to eat almost a whole box (six packs) in one sitting. She was also enjoying low-fat yogurt for an evening snack right before she went to bed. I told her that was good. She then asked me if having *three* of them at once was too much (as a snack). My silence told her yes.

My mother made a good effort to focus on lower-calorie and/or lower-fat foods. That was positive. What was not as good was the *quantity* of food she was eating. She was doing what many of us do:

eating too much of a good thing. Once she cut back her portions, she lost weight and her blood sugar and cholesterol levels improved.

Sometimes it's easy to make a fix, as in the case of my mother. She was eating the right things, just way too much of them. All she basically had to do was decrease her portion sizes. But while many eat the healthier packaged foods, a lot of us don't. Did you know that *one* Kellogg's Frosted Strawberry Pop Tart has 200 calories, 5 g of fat and 170 mg of sodium? And that a serving size is one Pop Tart, not two, as they're packaged? Because one package has two Pop Tarts, this probably leads many to consume both at one sitting for a total of 400 calories, 10 g of fat and 340 mg of sodium. How about the fact that 15 Lay's Classic Potato Chips contain 150 calories, 10 g of fat and 180 mg of sodium? Who eats only 15 chips? If you go to Subway and want chips, you can get them—the healthier kind. Subway sells individual-size bags of Baked Lays Potato Chips, which have 130 calories, 2 g of fat and 200 mg of sodium. This is a better choice, but it's important to note that there's a bit more sodium in the baked variety.

And of course, there are conventional sit-down chain restaurants, like Claim Jumper and Friday's, which now have offerings in the grocery store frozen food aisles. Two pieces of Friday's frozen Chicken Quesadilla Rolls will cost you 250 calories, 12 g of fat and 410 mg of sodium. If you like pizza, three of Totino's Ultimate Pepperoni Mega Pizza Rolls have 230 calories, 11 g of fat and 580 mg of sodium. We eat most of these types of food items as snacks, not as meals. Often we eat more than the one serving size indicated on the label.

Besides snacks, we also eat whole meals out of boxes, bags and cans. Many of these are loaded with calories and fat. For example, if you eat a Hungry-Man Boneless White Meat Fried Chicken frozen dinner, it will pack on 710 calories, 29 g, of fat and 2,160 mg of sodium. In this case, a visit to KFC could actually be the better choice.

I recently picked up a Pollo Bowl frozen entrée from El Pollo Loco, a fast food Mexican chain in nine U.S. states. For some reason, quite unlike me, I didn't check the nutrition facts label before I brought it home. Much to my dismay, I discovered that one bowl contained *two* servings. Had I not looked at the nutrition facts, I would've thought, as I'm sure many would, that one container would be one serving! One serving is 280 calories, 9 grams of fat and 960 mg of sodium. Eating the whole bowl, which isn't that big and which I'm sure a lot you would consume 560 calories, 18 grams of fat and 1,920 mg of sodium.

It's clear, then, that just like the many other accusations against the fast food corporations, rising obesity rates can't be entirely blamed on the industry. Home-cooked meals, just like sit-down restaurant offerings, are often loaded with calories and fat. It's important to consider what we eat, wherever we eat. As we'll see, it's a simple matter to incorporate fast food into a healthy lifestyle.

TWELVE

Factually Speaking

"There's quite a body of research out there that has proven no matter how you serve the food—whether in a bowl, a cup, a plate—the more you're served, the more you'll eat."

—Carolyn Dunn, PhD, North Carolina State University professor and nutrition specialist and chair of North Carolina's Eat Smart, Move More Initiative

As much as dietitians like to discuss fat, carbohydrate, protein and cholesterol, occasionally the key to good nutrition is much simpler. Sometimes it comes down to sheer quantity. At least part of the reason that sit-down restaurant menu items are often more caloric than their fast food counterparts is that they are often served in larger portions. With oversized meals, the overall nutrition content can also be worse. And studies have shown that when portion sizes are bigger, the majority will eat between 30 to 50 percent more food.

> David Zinczenko, editor-in-chief of Men's Health magazine notes the average meal at a sit-down restaurant is typically not as healthy as a similar meal at a fast food restaurant. With regard to sit-down restaurants, he concludes this type of eatery "is actually considerably worse for you than the often-maligned fast food fare. In fact, our menu analysis of 24 national chains revealed that the average entrée at a sit-down restaurant contains 867 calories, compared with 522 calories in the average fast food entrée. And that's before appetizers, sides or desserts – selections that can easily double your total calorie intake."

Some healthcare professionals have cited "unit bias" when it comes to the quantity of food we consume. This refers to a person's "psychological need," regardless of hunger, to eat whatever amount is served them. Nutrition specialist Carolyn Dunn, PhD, summed it up well when she said, "It doesn't matter how hungry you are or what you ate earlier. You generally eat more than you need to if it is put in front of you." And it's not so easy to combat this desire. "The battle against portion size is supersized," Dunn said. "People don't want to hear they need to step away from the table."

Studies have indicated that children eat close to double the amount of calories at a restaurant than they would at home (but that doesn't mean at-home eating is off the hook with regard to unhealthy and oversized portions). Other things such as fat, cholesterol, sodium and carbohydrate also increase and take residence in their bodies.

But be careful assuming which type of restaurant may contribute most to the excess weight on our children. A survey by the Center for Science in the Public Interest (CSPI) found that some sit-down restaurants serve up worse caloric/nutritional fare than fast food chains.

Some of the findings with regard to kid's meals were:

- The Applebee's grilled cheese sandwich had 520 calories and 14 g of saturated/trans fat. By adding fries to the sandwich, the calories totaled 900, equal to the saturated fat in three pork chops.
- The Boomerang cheeseburger with fries at Outback Steakhouse contained 840 calories and 31 g of saturated/trans fat, equivalent to eating a filet mignon, a sirloin steak and three butter pats. If the child rounded out the cheeseburger and fries with the Spotted Dog Sundae with chocolate sauce, he/she added 730 calories and 27 g of fat. The total meal would've been 1,700 calories and 58 g of saturated/trans fat.
- The Little Chicken Crispers at Chili's contained 360 calories and 8 g of saturated/trans fat. Adding fries brought the total count to 710 calories and 15 g of saturated/trans fat. This is the same amount of fat that would be consumed if the child ate two Quarter Pounders from McDonald's.

"Leave it to Chili's to turn a kid's meal into the nutritional equivalent of two adult-size burgers," said CSPI senior nutritionist Jayne G. Hurley. But it's important to note that both Chili's and Outback Steakhouse joined in the Kids LiveWell initiative with the goal of offering healthier meals to children.

We can and should navigate the waters of the restaurant menus and meals. It's not the restaurants' fault if we add on extra pounds. As Beth Bence Reinke, MS, RD, recently said, "Keep in mind that restaurants don't make people fat. It's what people choose to eat that causes weight gain. Each customer has complete freedom to make healthy choices or not. Every person who eats at restaurants frequently is not overweight, so there are ways to eat out without overdoing it." A sure fire way to do this is to read and understand the nutrition information that is provided.

The Facts

We know some restaurants with 20 or more locations must minimally provide total calories, saturated fat, carbohydrate and sodium for their menu items. This helps us make better choices. Many fast food restaurants go beyond that and give most or all of the information found on the nutrition facts labels of packaged products. This is fantastic. The more data, the better. Unfortunately, most of the affected sit-down restaurants aren't as comprehensive in their nutrition reporting.

> At the 2012 Olympics, McDonald's unveiled a nutrition QR code on its packaging. Customers can hold their smartphones up to it and get detailed nutrition information. This QR code will be available in the majority of McDonald's restaurants by 2013.

> Research has shown that the nutrition information at fast food restaurants may be more accurate than that provided at sit-down restaurants because fast food is more exactly portioned and usually served in standardized containers. At sit-down restaurants, the food is put on plates and the portion sizes may not be as well regulated.

But is providing the information enough? Do we know what it all means? Not everyone does. This is an area where all restaurants could step-up. Let's take a look at the nutrition information the restaurants provide. How does their food stack up?

Serving Size

Fast food restaurants and sit-down establishments will provide us with serving size information. All packaged, canned and bottled foods also give it. It's what the nutrition data is based on.

The serving sizes of packaged foods we find at coffeehouses and the like, artfully displayed near the register to tempt us as we pay for our lattes and cappuccinos, can also be an overindulgence. They're often larger than one serving size and much higher in calories than we should be consuming in a snack. In my lab coat I carry a small package of nuts and dried fruit from Starbucks, and I bring it out in most classes that I teach as an example of portion distortion and the very real need for reading nutrition facts labels. You might think the bag is one serving size and consume the whole thing along with your beverage. That would add 400 calories to the drink you're having, which, don't kid yourself, could also be a lot—up to 800 or more calories, depending on what you order and what you add to it. And if your beverage is on the higher- calorie end and you add in the bag of fruit and nuts, you wouldn't be far from consuming all the calories that you need in a day *in your snack*.

> A healthy plate contains fruits and vegetables on half of it, with protein and starch each taking one-quarter of the plate. Dairy is on the placemat.

Total Calories

Nutrition information provided by sit-down restaurants may not pertain to the entire meal. So read the fine print. Keep in mind if you want to lose weight, you need to reduce calories. One way to help do that is to take advantage of the calorie information that's provided. Numbers matter.

> The Oriental Grilled Chicken Salad at Applebee's has 1240 calories.
> The Sante Fe Chopped Salad at TGI Friday's contains 1,800 calories.
> The Premium Southwest Salad with Grilled Chicken at McDonald's has 290 calories.

The Fats

There are four types of fat, some of which are better for us than others: monounsaturated, polyunsaturated, saturated and trans fat. Heart-healthy fats like monounsaturated and polyunsaturated are the best way to go. However, remember that portion size counts. Gram for gram, fats have more than double the number of calories that carbohydrates and protein do. So fats, even healthier ones, are high in calories. They should be limited.

> The turkey burger at the sit-down restaurant Ruby Tuesday contains 18 more grams of fat than fast food restaurant Carl's Jr.'s turkey burger.

As a general rule, it's best to keep total fat intake to around 30 percent of total calories or less. Those with high cholesterol/heart disease might benefit from lower intakes of fat. Studies have shown that very low-fat diets (10 to 15 percent of total daily calories) can be effective in reversing heart disease.

A quick and easy way to keep total calories from fat in a healthy range is to look for three grams or less of total fat for every 100 calories. So if the item has 200 calories, aim for six grams or less of fat. If it has 300 calories, aim for nine grams or less of fat and so on.

Saturated Fat

Try to keep saturated fat intake to no more than 7 percent of total calorie intake. Saturated fats are usually solid at room temperature. Butter, milk, cheese, fatty cuts of meat and the skin of poultry are all saturated fats. So are coconut oil, palm oil and cocoa butter. Saturated fats can increase LDL ("bad" cholesterol) and can prompt the liver to make too much cholesterol. These aren't healthy choices.

Of the 80 grams of total fat in a half-rack of Outback's Baby Back Ribs, 30 grams are saturated. Not to be outdone, Denny's Grand Slamwich has 90 grams of total fat, of which 42 grams are saturated.

Unhealthy food choices can be found everywhere. A recent trend has been frying foods that aren't (and from a health perspective, shouldn't be) traditionally served fried. Fried ice cream has long been a staple at Mexican restaurants, but food carts (like one on the Las Vegas Strip) and state and county fairs have joined in on the frying fray. And boy, do we eat it up. All of these items have been served in a

cont. on page 162

cont. from page 161

weight- and artery-busting fried form: bubble gum, butter, Twinkies, Oreos, peanut butter and jelly sandwiches, Coca Cola, spaghetti and meatballs, jelly beans, pickles, bacon, cake, corn on the cob and cookie dough. You can also get a piece of fried chicken between two Krispy Kreme donuts.

Trans Fat

Trans fats are created through processing in which polyunsaturated fats are made to be solid at room temperature. This is called hydrogenation, and it's done to help increase the shelf life of products. So it's found in items such as margarine, lard, chips, crackers, cookies and ice cream. Look for the words "hydrogenated" or "partially hydrogenated." If you see them, keep away. The good news is that if you like margarine, there are many trans-fat free choices readily available.

Denny's Western Burger has 3 grams of trans fat. This may not sound like too much, but it is.

Cholesterol

We get cholesterol from two places, our livers and the food we eat. Most of us know we often get too much cholesterol from our diets. Unless a physician has told you otherwise, limit cholesterol to no more than 300 mg a day. For you bowlers, one way to remember this number is to think of that perfect game you may be striving for.

Where does cholesterol come from? If it has a face, a tail, feet/hooves, wings, gills, a head, a mother, a father, or comes from any of these things, then it contains cholesterol. Animals and animal products, in other words. If it comes from the ground, it doesn't contain cholesterol.

> Do you love those three egg omelets that you can get at a variety of sit-down restaurants? Depending on the size of the egg, the yolk could have between 200 and 250 mg of cholesterol. If you eat this omelet you would be ingesting close to three days-worth of cholesterol in one meal.

Total Sodium

I'm sad to say my husband is one of the many people who consume too much sodium. Sodium is a component of salt, and his MO is to salt his food before he even tastes it. I've asked him many times why he does this, and he always responds that he knows the food needs it. According to my husband, food can never be too salty.

When you think of sodium, picture it as a sponge. That is how it acts in our bodies, causing us to retain water. Why is this a problem? It makes our hearts work harder. For those with conditions such as congestive heart failure, this obviously isn't a good thing. Sodium can also increase our blood pressure, which, again, isn't good for our hearts.

Almost all restaurants do a terrible job on the sodium front. It's very difficult to find lower-sodium choices, but it's not impossible. Plain vegetables (10 mg a serving) and fruit (2 mg a serving) are examples of lower-sodium items. Every food has sodium, but some have sky-high amounts. The following looks at some restaurant offerings:

FAST FOOD VINDICATION

Restaurant	Menu Item	Sodium Content
Applebee's	Sizzling Skillet Fajitas - Steak	5,630 mg
	Quesadilla Burger	3,610 mg
California Pizza Kitchen	The Meat Cravers Pizza	4,163 mg
	Steak Tacos	1,423 mg
Claim Jumper	BBQ Chicken Sandwich	3,832 mg
	Frisco Burger	2,364 mg
Chili's	Boneless Buffalo Chicken Sandwich	4,330 mg
	Jalapeno Smokehouse Burger with Ranch Dressing	6,600 mg
Cheesecake Factory	Blackened Chicken Sandwich	2,440 mg
	The Club Sandwich	3,260 mg
Friday's	Japanese Hibachi Entrée—Grilled Chicken	4,720 mg
	Kansas City BBQ Burger	3,790 mg
Denny's	Double Cheeseburger	2,680 mg
	Spicy Buffalo Chicken Melt	3,760 mg
Burger King	Double Whopper	980 mg
	Spicy Chick'N Crisp Sandwich	810 mg
KFC	Spicy Crispy Chicken Breast	1,250 mg
	Popcorn Chicken— Large	1,480 mg
McDonald's	Angus Chipotle BBQ Bacon Sandwich	2,020 mg
	Big Mac	1,040 mg
Wendy's	Baconator Double	2,020 mg
	Asiago Ranch Chicken Club	1,630 mg
Taco Bell	XXL Grilled Stuft Burrito—Steak	2,050 mg
	Double Decker Taco	650 mg

Reviewing the table, we see that while both sit-down and fast food restaurants offer food that's high in sodium, the sit-down restaurants for the most part win the sodium sweepstakes with several items packed with 3,000 mg and up.

Carbohydrates

Carbohydrates turn very quickly into 100 percent sugar (glucose) in the blood. Sources include bread, pasta, rice, cereals, crackers, potatoes, corn, peas, beans, fruit/fruit juice and milk. They're an energy source and needed by our bodies, but monitoring portions is important. A serving size of rice or pasta is half of a cup or one-quarter of the plate. (For diabetics, it's a third of a cup.) I like to keep my serving sizes of carbohydrate to three to four servings a meal, about 45 to 60 grams of total carbohydrate. (One serving of carbohydrate is 15 grams.) This is also a good goal for diabetics. Check the nutrition information at the restaurants where you like to eat. Chances are your favorite entrées may have double, if not triple or more, grams of total carbohydrate in them. Doggie bags have never seemed more like a good thing, right?

Sit-down restaurants often give us far more carbohydrate than we should have in one meal. This includes carbs from pasta and rice. The amounts are off the chart. Take a look at the portion sizes of pasta at a few of the sit-down restaurants out there:

Restaurant	Portion Size of Spaghetti	# of ½ Cup Servings
California Pizza Kitchen	2 cups	4
Cheesecake Factory	4 cups	8
Claim Jumper	2.5 cups	5
Macaroni Grill	3.25 cups	6.5
Olive Garden	2 cups	4
Spumoni Italian Restaurant	4 cups	8

FAST FOOD VINDICATION

One of our favorite breakfast cereals is oatmeal, which is a starch. Starches are carbohydrates. A recommended serving size of cooked oatmeal is half of a cup. Here's how some of the restaurants stack up:

Restaurant	# of ½ Cup Servings of Oatmeal
Burger King	1
Coco's	2.25
IHOP	2.5
McDonald's	1

As you can see, the fast food restaurants give you an appropriate amount—one serving. The sit-down restaurants dish out over double the amount that's recommended.

Dietary Fiber

Plant foods such as grains, fruits, vegetables and legumes contain fiber. The body doesn't digest it. Fiber is good for you, but we all don't take advantage of this. It can help manage blood sugar, lower cholesterol, help with constipation, hemorrhoids, irritable bowel syndrome and diverticulosis. It can also keep you full, so it's helpful in weight-loss/weight-management efforts. It's recommended we get between 21 to 38 grams of fiber a day. The average person in America gets approximately 14 to 15 grams. While most people in the U.S. don't consume a lot of high-fiber foods, folks in other countries do. In China the average daily fiber intake is 77 grams.

> Look for cereals that have at least 5 grams of fiber in one serving. Oatmeal is one of them and there are also many cold cereals packed with fiber. Choosing low-fat/low-calorie toppings, if any, and monitoring portion size makes cereal a good choice at home and at restaurants.

Protein

A reasonable portion size of protein for lunch and dinner is 3 ounces (about 1 ounce for breakfast). Very often sit-down restaurants are the ones who "super-size" the burgers and other protein offerings. The following table takes a look at beef and turkey burgers. As you'll see, some of the "signature" fast food burgers (BK Whopper, Big Mac, Wendy's Single) are actually not oversized. This doesn't mean we can't get a larger burger at a fast food restaurant. Fatburger's XXXL 24-ounce burger is one. But it's difficult to find any sit-down restaurant hamburger that contains 3 ounces or less of protein. In fact, of the listed hamburgers, the fast food burger patties were all less than 3 ounces, while the patties at the sit-down restaurants all exceeded 3 ounces.

Restaurant Burger	Total Approximate Sandwich Weight	Approximate Meat Patty Weight	Does It Meet Portion Size Criteria?
Burger King Whopper (no cheese, no mayo)	9.8 ounces	2.8 ounces	Yes
Carl's Jr. Turkey Burger (no mayo)	7.9 ounces	2.9 ounces	Yes
Claim Jumper Hamburger (no cheese, no dressing)	11.6 ounces	4.4 ounces	No
Denny's Bacon Cheeseburger (no bacon, no cheese)	11.2 ounces	3.9 ounces	No
Island's Grill & Bar Big Wave Burger (no cheese)	11.5 ounces	3.9 ounces	No
McDonald's Big Mac (no cheese, no sauce)	5.7 ounces	2 ounces	Yes

Red Robin Gourmet Cheeseburger (no cheese, no mayo)	11.1 ounces	3.7 ounces	No
Salt Creek Grill Turkey Burger	11.0 ounces	4.8 ounces	No
Wendy's Single Hamburger (no cheese, no mayo)	7.4 ounces	2.9 ounces	Yes

If you haven't already been reading the nutrition information provided by restaurants, I hope you've decided to make it a part of your daily life. It helps us make decisions that affect our waistlines and our health. How can you go wrong there?

THIRTEEN

It Takes a Village

"Twenty years ago, you would have maybe 20 to 30 chews per bite of food. Today, food is so highly processed and so stimulating it goes down in a wash (of saliva), like we're eating adult baby food."

—Dr. David Kessler, professor at University of California San Francisco and former FDA commissioner

As much as we sometimes hate to hear it, we're ultimately responsible for ourselves—and that includes what we put in our mouths. While there may be obstacles in our way, it's up to us to figure out a way around them. The onus is also on us to mobilize those on our "team," such as family, friends and our health care providers. We're the CEOs of our health.

Given that, it's important that we get the information necessary to chart our healthy course. Knowledgeable people and entities can provide us with an arsenal of tools that we can draw from. Take advantage of what's already out there and spread the word to those in your sphere of influence. Here are some things I'd like to see happen to help us in that endeavor:

Change Is In the Air…If We Make It Happen

•   **Bring on the PSAs and Healthy Eating TV Segments**

I'm of an age that I remember the old public service announcements broadcast on TV in the evening. Who remembers the question, "It's 10 o'clock. Do you know where your children are?" Decades have passed and it still sticks in my mind. These messages can resonate. Consequently, I'd love to see PSAs with good nutrition messages, such as "Have you eaten fruit and vegetables today?" or "Did you watch your portion sizes today?" Celebrity spokespeople could make these even more effective, the strategy used successfully in the "Got Milk?" print ads.

I'd go even further with news programs including a healthy eating message at least once a week. It would be great to see similar segments on talk shows as well. While in school studying for my master's in nutritional science, I actually emailed *The Ellen DeGeneres Show* to suggest they consider including a monthly healthy cooking/ eating out segment. It could have been done in a humorous way. I'm quite certain Ellen gets a lot of mail, so I wasn't surprised when I heard nothing back. But how cool would that have been?

Sometimes celebrities use their influence for causes that are questionable. In early 2012, Wendy Williams, host of *The Wendy Williams Show*, embarked on a campaign to save the Twinkie from extinction when its maker, Hostess, filed for bankruptcy. She regularly promoted the spongy cream-filled cake, encouraged guests to talk about their memories and enjoyable moments involving Twinkies and other Hostess products, and gave them gifts of Twinkies. She hoped to ensure "our children and our children's children" will be able to consume "the golden symbol of the American dream." At 150 calories and 2.5 g of saturated fat a cake, this is certainly not one of the healthiest subjects of this kind of campaign.

> In Chapter 8, I highlight some of the charitable contributions and community benefit programs that fast food restaurants engage in. While I find this admirable, it would be great if these companies could channel some of that money into healthy eating advertisements and messages.

- **Explain the Information**

It's fantastic that we're provided with nutrition information on packaged foods and many restaurant menus. But I don't think that's enough. Facts and data don't impact us if we don't know what they mean. They need to be explained. I did just that in this book, but as much as I would love it if everyone in the world read this book, I know that's unlikely. So more needs to be done. Informational brochures in all restaurants and grocery stores would be a great step in this direction.

- **Expand the Information**

I would like to see all restaurants report nutrition information, regardless of their size. At the very least, lower the requirement to restaurants with three or even five or more locations instead of 20. Pictures of the USDA's My Plate somewhere on the menu as well as messages about the recommended amount of fruits, vegetables, dairy, grains and proteins to be eaten each day would be helpful.

- **Bring on the Healthy Cooking Shows**

We don't have many healthy cooking shows out there, so this is a niche ready to be carved out. I also suggest that all the cooking shows make an effort to include healthier recipes and discuss substitutions that would lighten up the concoctions they're creating. It would also be helpful if nutrition information were provided. And while I applaud Bobby Deen's show *Not My Mama's Meals* on the Cooking Channel, which lightens up Paula Deen's recipes, the Deen family and other celebrity chefs could do more.

- **Cookbooks and Magazines Should Step Up**

All cookbooks and magazines should provide nutrition information for every recipe they publish.

- **Expand or Introduce Nutrition Education in Schools and Centers**

In order to become a registered dietitian, I had to intern for a school year at a variety of different organizations. One of those stints was for Network for a Healthy California, which goes into schools for students of all ages and provides nutrition information through food demonstrations, exhibitions and games. It was very interesting and rewarding. My only suggestion would be to expand efforts to reach the parents and guardians of the younger kids, perhaps through PTA meetings, emails/mailers and after-school/evening classes/presentations.

> Michelle Obama's "Let's Move" campaign goal "to eliminate this problem of childhood obesity in a generation" takes good steps in this area by looking to improve food quality in schools, educate parents on nutrition and exercise, placing an emphasis on physical education, and working to get "affordable and accessible" nutritious foods for families.

- **Employers Should Get into the Wellness Business**

Many companies provide education and wellness programs already. My recommendation is that more get into the act. It can be as simple as bringing in a dietitian and/or exercise instructor to a staff meeting on a regular basis. Providing stress management coaching/techniques would also be helpful. After all, healthy, happy workers are more productive.

- **Keep It Going, Restaurants!**

Thank you for the healthier offerings. Please keep them on the menu and bring on more.

Conclusion

I speak to so many people in my professional capacity who are ready to make necessary changes to eat better and improve their health. I've also worked with some, despite their often critical health issues, who aren't anywhere close to change. That's to be expected.

Change can be hard. Many of us don't want to face it. Altering our habits, large or small, can be overwhelming. But many of us literally must change to survive. Start slowly and build your healthy lifestyle. And after reading this book, you should know now, if you didn't already, that fast food can be a part of that lifestyle.

I've always believed, and still do, that if I reach just one person with my message, then I've achieved success. That person will go on to influence others in his/her circle, and on and on it will go. That's how change happens.

It's my hope that my message has resonated with you, that I've answered some questions, and that you've created an action plan. I hope you have the tools to eat healthy, nutritious meals out and about, wherever you may find yourself, as you lead your life. It's clear that from fast food to fine dining, from vending machines to convenience stores, from farmers' markets and grocery stores to the kitchen table, it can be done.

So do it. Eat to live.

References

A Sabbath Blog. (2012, January 14). *ABC News features group of Adventists wanting to ban McDonald's in Loma Linda.* [Web log post]. Retrieved from http://www.asabbathblog.com/ 2012/01/ abc-news-features-group-of-adventists.html

Albright, C.L., Flora, J.A., & Fortman, S.P. (1990). Restaurant menu labeling: impact of nutrition information on entrée sales and patron attitudes [Abstract]. *Health Educ Q.* 17(2): 157-67. Abstract retrieved from http://www.ncbi.nlm.nih.gov/pubmed/

ALEC Exposed. (2008, August). *McDonald's.* Retrieved from http:// www.sourcewatch.org/ index.php?title=McDonald's

Aleccia, J. (2008, November). Rising risk for obese kids: Middle-aged arteries: Ultrasound imaging reveals accelerated evidence of heart disease. *NBC News.* Retrieved from http:// www.msnbc.msn.com/id/27651277/ns/health-health care/t/ rising-risk-obese-kids- middle-aged-arteries/

aliciadenney-g. (2006). Average fast food consumption per week. *Google Answers.* Retrieved from http://answers.google.com/ answers/threadview/id/779290.html

Aliday, E. (2011, December 8). Fast-food toy ban no aid to nutrition, study says. *San Francisco Chronicle.* Retrieved from http:// www.sfgate.com

Aliza. (2008, February 17). Obesity society's president protests menu labeling. *U.S. Food Policy.* Retrieved from http://usfoodpolicy. blogspot.com/2009/02/obesity-societys-president- protests.html

Altman, E.B., Fry, S. & Klinger, H. (2012, May). If things carry on this way, most adults will be obese by 2025. *Cooking Light Magazine.*

Amen, D. (2011, October 21). Holy unhealthy eating! How to stop churches from sending people to heaven early. [Web log post]. *Huffington Post.* Retrieved from http://www.huffingtonpost.com/ dr-daniel-amen/how-to-stop-churches-from_b_1021901.html

American Diebetes Association. & American Dietetic Association. (2008). *Choose your foods: Exchange lists for diabetes.* Alexandria, VA, Chicago IL.

American Dietetic Association. (2010, January). *Nutrition labeling of restaurant foods: An important piece of a broad vision for health reform.* [Electronic mailing list message].

American Dietetic Association. (2010, January). *Restaurant and packaged foods can have more calories than nutrition labeling indicates.* Retrieved from http://www.eatright.org/Media/ content. aspx?id=4294967696

American Red Cross. (2011). *Burger King Corp. to support American Red Cross emergency fleet.* Retrieved from http://redcross.org/

Amy T. (2012, January 3). Can you trust nutrition labels? [Web log post]. *Diabetes Mine.* Retrieved from http://www.diabetesmine. com/2012/01/can-you-trust-nutrition-labels.html

Anderson, D. (2008, May). Eating out in America: A new war wages. *Nielson Consumer Insight Magazine.* Retrieved from http://www. nielsen.com/consumer_insight/issue8/ci_topline_articleV11.html

Andrews, W. (2011, February). 'Tsunami' of obesity worldwide: study. *Yahoo! News.* Retrieved from http://news.yahoo.com/s/ afp/20110204/hl_afp/healthscienceobesity_20110204023011

Answers.com. (n.d.). *Burger King corporation.* Retrieved August 25, 2008 from http://www.answers.com/topic/burger-king

AP. (2008, October 7). McDonald's seeks retirees to fill void. *The New York Times.* Retrieved from http://query.nytimes.com/

AP News. (2012, June). Krispy Kreme inks deal to open 80 stores in India. *Bloomberg Businessweek.* Retrieved from http://www.businessweek.

com/ap/2012-06-13/krispy-kreme- inks-deal-to-open-80-stores-in-india

Applebee's. (2012). *Nutritional information.* Retrieved from http://www.applebees.com/~/media/docs/Applebees Nutritional Info.ashx

Associated Press. (2003, November). McDonald's not lovin 'McJob' dictionary definition. *CNN.* Retrieved from http://www.cnn.com/

Associated Press. (2005, January). McDonald's 'obesity' lawsuit back in court. *Newsmax.* Retrieved from http://archive.newsmax.com/archives/articles/2005/1/26/101537.shtml

Associated Press. (2005, August). Woman says 'McDonald's diet' took off weight. *MSNBC.* Retrieved from http://www.msnbc.msn.com/id/8916080/

Associated Press. (2005, August). Woman loses weight on McDonald's-only diet. *CTV.ca.* Retrieved from http://www.ctv.ca/servlet/ArticleNews/story/CTVNews/1123889717433 9/?hub=Health

Associated Press. (2007, February). Obese British boy will stay with mom. *NBC News.* Retrieved from http://www.msnbc.com/id/17366915/ns/health-kids and parenting/

Associated Press. (2008, July). Los Angeles bans fast food restaurants in poorer areas. *The Raw Story.* Retrieved from http://rawstory.com/news/2008/Los Angeles bans fast food restaurants 0729.html

Associated Press. (2009, May). Fugitive mom, 555-pound son found in Md. *MSNBC.* Retrieved from http://www.msnbc.msn.com/id/30877017/ns/us news-crime and courts/

Associated Press. (2010, February). First lady begins fight against childhood obesity. *Yahoo! News.* Retrieved from http://news.yahoo.com/s/ap/20100209/ap on go pr wh/us michelle obama obesity

Associated Press. (2010, March 3). Anger over Weight Watchers' endorsement of McDonald's. *The Guardian.* Retrieved from http://www.guardian.co.uk/

Associated Press. (2010, September). McDonald's denies report of dropping healthcare. *Yahoo! Finance.* Retrieved from http://finance.yahoo.com/news/McDonalds-denies-report-of-apf-455701319.html?x=0

Associated Press. (2011, July). Study: NYC fast-food menu calorie counts work for some. *USA Today.* Retrieved from http://yourlife.usatoday.com/

Associated Press. (2011, November 28). Ohio puts 200-pound third-grader in foster care. [Web log post]. *The Plain Dealer. USA Today.* Retrieved from http://yourlife.usatoday.com/

Bad habits: Poor diet, smoking, drinking, sloth can age you 12 years. (2010, April 26). *USA Today.* Retrieved from http://www.usatoday.com/

Baertlein, L. (2011, April 4). McDonald's plans to add 50,000 jobs on 'hiring day.' Retrieved from http://www.huffingtonpost.com/

Baertlein, L. (2011, July 7). Mississippi most obese state, Colorado least. *Reuters.* Retrieved from http://www.reuters.com/article/2011/07/07/us-usa-obesity-idUSTRE7663JD20110707

Baertlein, L. (2011, November.) McDonald's toy sale skirts Happy Meal restrictions. *Reuters.* Retrieved from http://news.yahoo.com/mcdonald's-toy-sale-skirts-happy-meal-restrictions-012637382.html

Baguio, L. (2009, February, 6). Ronald McDonald room renovation aims to provide comfort. *The Orange County Register.* Retrieved from http://www.ocregister.com

Bakalar, N. (2010, January 11). Counting of calories isn't always accurate. *The New York Times.* Retrieved from http://www.nytimes.com/2010/01/12/health/12calo.html

balisunset. (n.d.). *Employees and employement in fast food industry.* Retrieved October 18, 2008 from http://hubpages.com/hub/Employees-and-employement-in-fast-food-industry

Barlow, T. (2010, January). *Study finds lite restaurant meals pack more calories than stated.* Retrieved from http://www.walletpop.com

Barrow, B. (2012, July 23). Forget McJobs – now you can take away a KFC degree: Fast food giant launches three-year business studies course. *Daily Mail Online*. Retrieved from http://www.dailymail.co.uk/

Bauman, V. (2005, August 14). McDonald's diet a growing trend. *Nashua Telegraph*. Retrieved from http://www.nashuatelegraph.com

Bergold, R. (2010, April). The nutrition-labeling mandate won't work unless a standard system is created to assign calorie counts. *QSR Magazine*. Retrieved from http://www.2.qsrmagazine.com/articles/columnists/_roy-bergold/0410/justthefacts-1.phtml

Berlin, L. (2011, July). McDonald's Happy Meals get a healthier overhaul. *Daily Finance*. Retrieved from http://www.dailyfinance.com/2011/07/26/mcdonalds-happy-meals-get-a-more-_healthy-overhaul/

Berr, J. (2010, June). Health groups says it will sue McDonald's over Happy Meals. *Daily Finance*. Retrieved from http://www.dailyfinance.com/2010/10/06/health-group-says-it-will-sue-mcdonalds-over-happy-meals/

Berr, J. (2010, July). Want a lawsuit with that? McDonald's defends Happy Meal marketing. *Daily Finance*. Retrieved from http://www.dailyfinance.com/2010/07/21/want-a-lawsuit-_with-that-mcdonalds-defends-happy-meal-marketin/

Betsy. (2011, January 11). *Sign of times to come: California state law goes into effect (sort of)*. Retrieved from http://menutrinfo.com/2011/01/11/sign-times-california-state-law-effect-sort/

BETT Middle East. (2008, November). *McDonald's Bahrain marks world children's day with memorable celebration*. Retrieved from http://www.ameinfo.com/176750.html

Better Business Bureau. (2008). *Ronald McDonald House Charities*. Retrieved from http://charityreports.bbb.org/Public/Report.aspx?CharityID=195

Big soda ban proposed by mayor of Cambridge, Mass. (2012, June). *CBS News*. Retrieved from http://www.cbsnews.com/8301-504763_162-57456252-10391704/big-soda-ban-proposed-by-_mayor-of-cambridge-mass/

Biggs, F. (Ed.). (2007) *Simple essential family favorites: Over 500 delicious step-by-step recipes.* Bath, UK: Parragon Books Ltd.

Bittman, M. (2009). *Food matters: A guide to conscious eating.* New York, NY: Simon & Schuster Paperbacks.

BK Worldwide. (2008). *Minority organizations.* Retrieved from http://bk.com/companyinfo/ diversity/minority.aspx

Block, J.P., Scribner, R.A., & DeSalvo, K.B. (2004). Fast food, race/ethnicity, and income a geographic analysis. *Am J Prev Med,* 27(3), 211-217.

Bly, L. (2012, April 24). Another patron collapses at Vegas' Heart Attack Grill. *USA Today.* Retrieved from http://www.usatoday.com/

Bly, L. (2012, June 1). Will tourists swallow a NYC ban on supersize sugary drinks? *USA Today.* Retrieved from http://www.usatoday.com/

Bob Evans. (2012). Nutrition information for Bob Evans menu items. Retrieved from http://www.bobevans.com/Menu/Nutritional-Information

Bob Greene renews 'go active' relationship with McDonald's. (2005, January). *QSR Magazine.* Retrieved from http://www.qsrmagazine.com/articles/news/story.phtml?id=4391

bon appetite. (2009, September).

Bonisteel, S. (2009, August 7). PETA unhappy meals targeting kids. *Slashfood.* Retrieved from http://www.slashfood.com

Borland, S. (2012, July 17). Why being a couch potato is as bad for you as smoking: Failing to get fit causes 90,000 deaths a year. *Daily Mail.* Retrieved from http://www.dailymail.co.uk/

Bove fined for GM crop rampage. (2002, October). *BBC News.* Retrieved from http://news.bbc.co.uk/1/hi/world/europe/2351191.stm

Bowman, S.A., Gortmaker, S.L., Ebbeling, C.B., Pereira, M.A., & Ludwig, D.S. (2004). Effects of fast-food consumption on energy intake and diet quality among children in a national household survey. *Pediatrics,* 113(1), 112-118. Retrieved from http://pediactrics.aapublications.org/cgi/content/abstract/113/1/112

Bowman, S.A. & Vinyard, B.T. (2009). A look at how fast food affects U.S. adults: Impact on energy nutrient intake and over-weight status. *J Am Coll Nutr,* 23, 163-168. Retrieved from http://www.diabetes.org/diabetes-research/summaries.bowman-fastfood.jsp

Boy, you are one big baby! Lu Hao, the three-year-old who weighs a staggering 132lbs – and he's still growing. (2011, March 23). *Daily Mail Reporter.* Retrieved from http://www.daily-mail.co.uk/news/article-1368790/Lu-Hao-Chinese-toddler-3-weighs-staggering-132lbs-hes-growing.html

Brandau, M. (2012, April). NRA: Restaurant industry posts significant job growth. *National Restaurant Association.* Retrieved from http://nrn.com/article/nra-restaurant-industry-posts- significant-job-growth

Brandi. (2010, February 9). Michelle Obama launches childhood obesity intiative with LetsMove.Gov. *Diets in Review.* Retrieved from http://www.dietsinreview.com/diet_column/02/michelle-obama-launches-childhood-obesity-initiative-with-letsmove-gov/

Brandon, E. (2010, March 22). 30 fast-growing careers for older workers – planning to retire. *U.S. News.* Retrieved from http://money.usnews.com/

Brassfield, M. (2011, January). Big-city fast-food bans: the Los Angeles ban on new fast food restaurants in South L.A. takes on obesity. *CalorieLab.* Retrieved from http://calorielab.com/news/2011/01/16/los-angeles-ban-on-new-fast-food-restaurants/

Briggs, H. (2011, June). Snacking clue to obesity epidemic. *BBC News.* Retrieved from http://www.bbc.co.uk/news/health-13948071

British officials may take custody of extremely overweight boy. (2007, March 15). *USA Today.* Retrieved from http://www.usa-today.com/

Brown, C. (2008, January 29). Teachers furious at plans for 'McDonald's diplomas.' *The Independent.* Retrieved from http://www.independent.co.uk/

Brownell, K.D., & Battle Horgen, K. (2004). *Food fight: The inside story of the food industry, America's obesity crisis & what we can do about it.* New York, NY: McGraw-Hill.

Buchholz, T.G. (2003). *Fast food is not the primary cause of obesity.* Collins, T. B. (Ed.), *Fast food.* Farmington Hills, MI: Thomson Gale.

Buhi, L.K. (n.d.) *Food insecurity.* Retrieved October 30, 2008 from http://www.faqs.org/nutrition/Erg-Foo/Food-Insecurity.html

Bumgardner, W. (2009, March 10). Bob Greene walks and bikes across the USA. McDonald's Go active American challenge 2004. *About.com Walking.* Retrieved from http://walking.about.com/cs/longdistance/a/greenegoactive.htm

Burbach, K. (2004, December). Swarts helped bring Ronald McDonald House to Omaha. *UNMC today.* Retrieved from http://app.1.unmc.edu/publicaffairs/todaysite/sitefiles/today_full.cfm?match=1943

Bureau of Labor Statistics. (2002). *Declining teen labor force participation.* Retrieved from http://www.bls.gov/opub/ils/pdf/opbils49.pdf

Bureau of Labor Statistics. (2007a). *Occupational employment statistics. Occupational employment and wages, May 2007, waiters and waitresses.* Retrieved from http://www.bls.gov/OES/current/oes353031.htm

Bureau of Labor Statistics. (2007b). *Occupational employment statistics. Occupational employment and wages, May 2007, cooks, fast food.* Retrieved from http://www.bls.gov/OES/current/oes352011.htm

Bureau of Labor Statistics. (2007c). *Occupational employment statistics. May 2007 national industry-specific occupational employment and wage estimates, full-service restaurants.* Retrieved from http://www.bls.gov/OES/current/naics4_722100.htm

Bureau of Labor Statistics. (2008a). *Employment status of the civilian population by sex and age.* Retrieved from http://www.bls.gov/news.release/empsit.t01.htm

Bureau of Labor Statistics. (2008b). *Employment situation summary.* Retrieved from http://www.bls.gov/news.release/empsit.nr0.htm

Bureau of Labor Statistics. (2008c). *Older workers. Are there more older people in the workplace.* Retrieved from http://www.bls.gov/spotlight/2008/older_workers/

Burger King. (2008a). *Burger King/Mclamore Foundation and United Negro College Fund – a winning combination for higher education.* Retrieved from http://www.bk.com/companyinfo/content/community/nr05152006.html

Burger King. (2008b). *Burger King scholars program.* Retrieved from http://www.bk.com/company/info/community/BKS.aspx

Burger King. (2008c). *Community outreach.* Retrieved from http://www.bk.com/companyinfo/ community.aspx?target=main

Burger King. (2008d). *Diversity action council.* Retrieved from http://www.bk.com/companyinfo/diversity/dac.aspx

Burger King. (2008e). *Burger King employee scholars program.* Retrieved from http://www.bk.com/companyinfo/community/BKES.aspx

Burger King. (2008f). *Together we can.* Retrieved from http://www.bk.com/companyinfo/ diversity/community.aspx

Burger King. (2012). *Menu and Nutrition.* Retrieved from http://www.bk.com/en/us/menu- nutrition/index.html

Burton, S., Creyer, E.H, Kees, J., & Huggins, K. (2006). Attacking the obesity epidemic: The potential health benefits of providing nutrition information in restaurants. *American Journal of Public Health*, 96 (9). Retrieved from http://web.ebscohost.com.mimas.calstatela.edu/

Business & Legal Reports. (2001, July). *Supersizing fast-food jobs with benefits.* Retrieved from http://compensation.blr.com/display.cfm/id/150637

Business Civic Leadership Center. (2011). *Corporate aid tracker – Japanese earthquake and tsunami.* Retrieved from http://bclc.uschamber.com/site-page/corporate-aid-tracker-japanese-earthquake-and-tsunami-march-2011

California Center for Public Health Advocacy. (2008). *Implementation of SB 1420: What it means for California communities.* Retrieved from http://www.publichealthadvocacy.org

California Center for Public Health Advocacy. (2009). *Resources: menu labeling.* Retrieved from http://www.publichealthadvocacy.org/resources_menulabeling.html

California Conference of Directors of Environmental Health., California Department of Public Health., California Restaurant Association., California Retailers Association., California Hotel and Lodging Assocation., et al. (2009). *California menu labeling guidelines July 2009.*

California Pizza Kitchen. (n.d.). *Nutritional Menu Guide.*

California Restaurant Association. (n.d.). *Overview of California's menu labeling law. Food facilities affected by the California menu labeling law.* Retrieved from http://www.calrest.org/issues-policies/key-issues/health-nutrition/menu-labeling/overview-ca- menu-labeling-law/

Campbell's. (2006). *Casseroles, one-dish meals and more.* Lincolnwood, IL: Publications International Ltd.

Cantalupo's response to Merriam Webster's definition of McJobs earns praise. (2003, November). *QSR Magazine.* Retrieved from http://m.qsrmagazine.com/news/ cantalupo-s-response-merriam-webster-s-definition-mcjobs-earns-praise

Carbone, N. (2011, September). The most creative (and ridiculous) state fair food: Fried bubble gum. *News Feed.* Retrieved from http://newsfeed.time.com/2011/09/06/the-most-creative- and-ridiculous-state-fair-food-fried-bubble-gum/

Carl's Jr. (2012). *Nutrition information.* Retrieved from http://www.carlsjr.com/system /pdf_menus/20/original/05012012_CKE_nutcalc_cvr_nutritionguide_nogb COMBINE[3].pdf?1335923480

Carl Karcher Enterprises, Inc. (2008). *The Carl's Jr. story.* Retrieved from http://www.carlsjr.com/company/story/

Carlino, B., Stefanelli, J., & Pavesic, D.V. (1989, May). Hiring the handicapped. *Nation's Restaurant News.* Retrieved from http://findarticles.com/p/articles/mi_m3190/is_/ai_7633767

Carnia, C. (2012, June 1). Boehner to Bloomberg: Super size me on that soda. *USA Today.* Retrieved from http://content.usatoday.com/

Carroll, B. (2010). McDonald's connects with employees and customers. *Amazing Service Guy.* http://amazingserviceguy.com

Cassady, D., Housemann, R., & Dagher, C. (2004). Measuring cues for health choices on on restaurant menus: development and testing of a measurement instrument [Abstract]. *Am J Health Promot.* Abstract retrieved from http://www.ncbi.nlm.nih.gov/pubmed/

Catalyst. (2011). *Catalyst honors initiatives at Kaiser Permanente, McDonald's Corporation, and Time Warner Inc. with the 2011 catalyst award.* Retrieved from http://www.catalyst.org/press-release/182/catalyst-honors-initiatives-at-kaiser-permanente-mcdonalds-corporation-and-time-warner-inc-with-the-2011-catalyst-award

CDC. (n.d.). *Behavioral risk factor surveillance system.* Retrieved from http://www.cdc.gov/brfss/

CDC. (n.d.). *Frequently asked questions about calculating obesity-related risk.* Retrieved from http://www.cdc.gov/PDF/Frequently Asked Questions About Calculating Obesity-Related_risk.pdf

CDC. (2008). *U.S. obesity trends 1985-2007.* Retrieved from http://www.cdc.gov/nccdphp /dnpa/obesity/trend/maps/index.htm

Cederquist, C.J. (2009) Eating healthy restaurant dining out, weighing in: Restaurant meals are higher in calories. *Bistro M.D.* Retrieved from http://www.bistromd.com/eatinghealth restaurant.asp

Centers for Disease Control and Prevention. (2007a). *Fruit and vegetable consumption among adults ---United States,* 2005. Retrieved from http://www.cdc.gov/mmwR/preview/mmwrhtml/mm5610a2.htm

Centers for Disease Control and Pevention. (2007b). *Prevalence of regular physical activity among adults –United States 2001 and 2005.*

Retrieved April 16, 2008 from http://www.cdc.gov/mmwr/preview/mmwrhtml/mm5646al.htm?s_cid=mm5646a1.e

Centers for Disease Control and Prevention. (2008). *Overweight and Obesity.* Retrieved from http://www.cdc.gov/nccdphp/dnpa/obesity/

Centers for Disease Control and Prevention. (2011). *Americans consume too much sodium (salt).* Retrieved from http://www.cdc.gov/features/dsSodium/

Center for Science in the Public Interest. (2003). *NY state menu labeling bill introduced: Legislation would put nutrition info on chain restaurant menus, menu boards.* Retrieved from http://www.cspinet.org/new/200303111.html

Cevallos, M. (2011, April 21). Dieters find 'healthy' food labels can be tricky. *Los Angeles Times.* Retrieved from http://articles.latimes.com/

CFIF. (2005, January). *Reheating a deep fried cause.* Retrieved from www.cfif.org/htdocs/legal issues/...cases/mcdonalds-lawsuit.htm

Chan, A. (2011, July 26). McDonald's Happy Meals to get less fries, more fruit. *The Huffington Post.* Retrieved from http://www.huffingtonpost.com/2011/07/26/mcdonalds-happy-meal-apples_n_909605.html?

Chan, A.L. (2012, July 19). Physical inactivity responsible for nearly 1 out of every 10 deaths around the world: study. Retrieved from http://www.huffingtonpost.com/

Chan, S. (2002, July). 'Food court' takes on new meaning: Man sues fast food chains over his_ health problems. *CBS News.* Retrieved from http://www.cbsnews.com/stories/2002/08/28/ health/main520007.shtml

Chandon, P. & Wansink, B. (2007). The biasing health halos of fast-food restaurant claims. *Cornell University Food and Brand Lab.* Retrieved from http://foodpsychology.cornell.edu/outreach/health-halos.html

Chang, A. (2011, June 23). Potato chips worst culprit for weight gain. *USA Today.* Retrieved from http://yourlife.usatoday.com/

Chapman, S. (2008, February). A tick for Macca's, but is your ticker the winner? *Smh.com*. Retrieved from http://www.smh.com.au/news/

Chasick, A.(2009, June). Oregon set to require menu labeling for chain restaurants. *Consumerist*. Retrieved from http://consumerist.com/5275658/

Cheesecake factory calorie counter. (2012). *Calorie Lab*. Retrieved from http://calorielab.com/news/2007/07/28/calorie-pusher-comes-to-town-the-cheesecake-factory- hits-rochester/

Chen, S. (2010, July). Cooking fries? Cleaning hospitals? Executives reflect on their first job. *CNN.com*. Retrieved from http://www.cnn.com/2010/LIVING/07/29/ceo.first.job.success /index.html

Child, J, Bertholle, L. & Beck, S. (2009). *Mastering the art of French cooking*. New York, NY: Alfred A. Knopf.

Chili's. (2012). *Nutrition*. Retrieved from http://www.brinker.com/gr/nutritional/chilis nutrition menu.pdf

Cheeseburger bill' puts bite on lawsuits. (2005, October). *CNN Politics*. Retrieved from chains-food-industry? s=PM:POLITICS

Chu, K. (2012, February 27). Yum Brands CEO takes on the world – a bite at a time. *USA Today*. Retrieved from http://usatoday.com

Claim Jumper. (2012). *Nutritional infromation*. Retrieved from http://www.claimjumper.com/menu nutritional information. aspx

CNN Money. (2011). World's most admired companies. *Fortune*. Retrieved from http://money.cnn/magazines/fortune/mostadmired/2011/full list/

Coco's Bakery. (n.d.). *Coco's menu nutritionals for website*. Retrieved from http://www.cocosbakery.com/wp-content/themes/cocos/pdf/nutritional-information.pdf

Cohen, A. (2011, July). States fight back against city laws on unhealthy food. *TIME*. Retrieved from http://www.time.com/time/nation/article/0,8599,2083685,00.html

Confessions of a Drive-Thru Runner. (n.d.). [Web log post]. Retrieved from http://mcrunner.com /?page_id=29

Conley, M. (2011, November). McDonald's skirts ban; charges 10 cents per Happy Meal toy. *ABC News*. Retrieved from http://abcnews.go.com/blogs/health/medical/unit/

Cottrell, M. (2011, January 19). City bans fast food restaurants. Should Chicago be next? *The Chicago Reporter*. Retrieved from http://www.chicagonow.com/

Courts charge mother of 555-pound boy. (n.d.). *ABC News*. Retrieved from http://abcnews.go._com/Health/WellnessNews/story?id=7941609

Critzer, G. (2003). *Fat land*. New York, NY: Houghton Mifflin Company.

Crowe, A. (2010, July). *Flipping burgers leads to fulfilling careers*. Retrieved from http://jobs.aol.com/articles/2010/07/09/restaurant-jobs/

Cusolito, N. (2011, April). On national hiring day, Staten Island McDonald's looking to beef up its staff. *SILive.com*. Retrieved from http://www.silive.com/northshore/index.ssf/2011/04 /on_national_hiring_day_staten.html

Daniels, C., Hickman, J (List), Chen, C.Y., Harrington, A., Lustgarten, A., Mero, J., & Tkaczyk, C. (Text). 50 best companies for minorities in an ideal world leading companies for minority employees would be tops for everyone. But this is not an ideal world, and some companies are still more successful at fostering diversity in their workplace than others. The good news: Corporate America is raising the bar, and the best keep on getting better. FORTUNE's list shows which 50 companies rank at the very top. *Fortune*. Retrieved from http://money.com.cnn.com/magazines/fortune/fortune_archive/2004/06/28/374393/index.htm

Dave Thomas Foundation for Adoption. (2008a). *Welcome to the Dave Thomas Foundation for adoption*. Retrieved from http://www.davethomasfoundation.org/

Dave Thomas Foundation for Adoption (2008b). *Wendy's wonderful kids.* Retrieved from http://www.davethomasfoundation.org/Our-Work/Wendy-s-Wonderful-Kids

Dave Thomas Foundation for Adoption. (2008c). *Wendy's wonderful kids marks 500th adoption.* Retrieved from http://www.davethomasfoundation.org/News?Wendy-s-Wonderful-Kids- Marks-500th-Adoption

Dave Thomas Biography. (2008d). *"Only in America."* Retrieved from http://wendys.com/

Davidson, P. (2011, September 5). Summer ends on sour note for jobless teens. *USA Today.* Retrieved from http://www.usatoday.com/

Davis, A. (2008, October 29). Boy aged six is among seven obese children taken into care. *Daily Mail.* Retrieved from http://www.dailymail.co.uk

Deardorff, J. (2007, June 6). Are heelys really dangerous? [Web log post]. *Chicago Tribune.* Retrieved from http://featuresblogs.chicagotribune.com/

Death, destruction, charity, salvation, war, money, real estate, spouses, babies, and other September 11 statistics. *New York Magazine.* Retrieved from http://nymag.com/news/articles/wtc/1year/numbers.htm

Deen, Paula (ed.) (n.d.). *Paula Deen's Best Dishes.* Birmingham, AL: Hoffman Media, LLC.

Denny's. (2012). *Nutrition menu.* Retrieved from http://www.dennys.com/files/nutrition_facts.pdfhttp://www.dennys.com/files/nutrition_facts.pdf

Denver, Kusa. (2012, March 9). 'Pink slime' eliminated from fast food, but not school lunches. *USA Today.* Retrieved from http://yourlife.usatoday.com

Dermody, C. (2010, May). KFC's double down is health! (uh compared to these meals...). *Shine from yahoo!* ®. Retrieved from http://shine.yahoo.com/channel/food/kfcs-double-down-is-healthy-uh-compared-to-these- meals-1366841.html

DeSorbo, M.A. (n.d.). Redefining the salad. *QSR Magazine*. Retrieved from http://www2.qsrmagazine.com/articles/features/120/salad-1.phtml

Diemer, T. (2011, February). Rush Limbaugh calls Michelle Obama 'hypocrite' for eating ribs. *Politics Daily*. Retrieved from http://www.politicsdaily.com/2011/02/22/rush-limbaugh-calls-michelle-obama-hypocrite-for-eating-ribs/

Diliberti, N., Bordi, P.L, Conklin, M.T., Roe, L.S., & Rolls, B.J. (2004). Increased portion size leads to increased energy intake in a restaurant meal. *Obesity Research*, 12, 562-568. Retrieved from http://www.obesityresearch.org/cgi/content/full/12/3/562.

Doell, L. (2010, November). San Francisco board overrides veto of happy meal toy ban. *Walletpop*. Retrieved from http://wallet-pop.com/

Don Gorske eats 25,000[th] Big Mac. (n.d.). *ABC News*. Retrieved from http//abcnews.go.cm/ health/don-gorske-wisconsin-eats-25000th-big-mac/story?id=13632899

Donation Doubler. (2011). *Mark Wahlberg & Taco Bell foundation for teens team up to fight high school dropout crisis.* Retrieved from http://donationdoubler.org/?p=549

Donkersloot, M. (1992). *The fast-food diet, quick and healthy eating at home and on the go.* New York, NY: Fireside, Simon and Schuster.

Donnelly, E. (2008, November). I'll take the 800-calorie cheesesteak: Philly's new menu- labeling laws. *Lemondrop*. Retrieved from http://www.lemondrop.com

Douglas, L. (2011, April). A year later, FDA proposes menu labeling requirements. *Serious Eats*. Retrieved from http://www.seriouseats.com/2011/04/calorie-counts-starbucks-fast-food- menu-labeling-fda.html

Dovarganes, Damian. (2012, March 6). Convenient cupcake dispensers are dangerous for dieters. *USA Today*. Retrieved from http://yourlife.usatoday.com

Duke Medicine News and Communications. (2004). *Modest exercise can prevent weight gain.* Retrieved from http://www.dukehealth.org/HealthLibrary/News/7325

Dunn, K. (2008, May 21). Can this turnover number from McDonald's (44%) be right? Retrieved from http://www.fistfuloftalent.com/2008/05/can-this-turnov.html.

Eater. (2008). *Fast food ban.* Retrieved from http://la.eater.com/tags/fast-food-ban.

Ebbeling, C.B., Sinclair, K.B., Pereira, M.A., Garcia-Lago, E., Feldman, H.A. & Ludwig, D.S. (2004). Compensation for energy intake from fast food among overweight and lean adolescents. *JAMA.* (291), 2828-2833. Retrieved from http://jama.ama-assn.org/cgi/content /full/291/23/2828

Edelbaum, M. (n.d.). The fast food ban. *Eating Well.* Retrieved from http://www.eatingwell.com/food_news_origins/food_news/the_fast_food_ban

Edwards, M. (2010, January). *Are misleading nutrition labels making you fat?* Retrieved from http://www.thatsfit.com/2010/01/08/are-misleading-nutrition-labels-making-you-fat/

Elan, E. (2008, April). Lottery winner says millions not enough; he's happiest working at McDonald's. *Nation's Restaurant News.* Retrieved from http://findarticles.com/p/articles/ mi_m3190/is_14_42/ai_n25356104/?tag=rel.res4

Ellis, J. (2012, January 9). Companies score foods' nutrition for grocers. *USA Today.* Retrieved from http://www.usatoday.com/

Environmental Working Group. (2011, December). *Kids' cereals pack more sugar than Twinkies and cookies.* Retrieved from http://www.ewg.org/release/kids-cereals-pack-more- sugar-twinkies-and-cookies

Eskenazi, J. (2011, November 29). Happy Meal ban: McDonald's outsmarts San Francisco. [Web log post]. *SF Weekly.* Retrieved from http://blogs.sfweekly.com/thesnitch/2011/11/happy_meal_ban_mcdonalds_outsm.php

Farfan, B. (2011). 2011 most admired retailers on Fortune "top 50 most admired companies" list. *About.com.* Retrieved from http://retailindustry.about.com/

Fast food facts from the Super Size Me web site. (n.d.). Retrieved August 25, 2008 from http://www.vivavegie.org/101book/text/nolink/social/supersizeme.htm

Fast food named one of the fastest growing industries.(2008, October). *QSR Magazine.* Retrieved from http://www.qsrmagazine.com/articles/news/story.phtml?id=6437

Ferguson, J.L. (2005, October). Teens, jobs and school: the pros and cons. *Ezine Articles.* Retrieved from http://ezinearticles.com/?Teens,-Jobs-and-School:-The-Pros-and-Cons& id=86750

Fernandez, M. (2006, September 24). Pros and cons of a zoning diet: Fighting obesity by limiting fast-food restaurants. *The New York Times.* http://www.nytimes.com/

Ferrin, L. (2010, February). Michelle Obama: 'Let's move' initiative battles childhood obesity. *ABC News.* Retrieved from http://abcnews.go.com/GMA/Health/michelle-obama-childhood- obesity-initiative/story?id=9781473

Fickenscher, L. (2009, November). Houston's restaurant outsmart calorie cops. *Crain's New York Business.* Retrieved from http://www.crainsnewyork.com/article/20091108/SUB /311089984

Fitzpatrick, M.P., Chapman, G.E., & Barr, S.I. (1997). Lower-fat menu items in restaurants satisfy customers [Abstract]. *Am Diet Assoc.* 97(5), 510-4. Abstract retrieved from http://www.ncbi.nlm.nih.gov/pubmed/

Flavelle, C. (2008, July). Super-vise me: It's ok to feel guilty about eating fast food, but is it the government's job? *Slate Magazine.* Retrieved from http://www.slate.com/id/2194629/ pagenum/all/

Flegal, K.M., Carroll, M.D., Ogden, C.L., & Johnson, C.L. (2002). Prevalence and trends in obesity among US adults, 1999-2000. *JAMA*, 288, 1723-1726.

Fogelholm, M., & Kukkonan-Hajula. (2001). A 10 year observational study found that girls who were not active during adolescence gained on average between 10 to 15 more pounds than girls who were active. *Obesity Reviews.* 1(2), 95-111.

Food Awareness. (2012). *Longevity.* Retrieved from http://fooda-wareness.org/life_span_11.html

Food Network Magazine. (2009, October.).

Frame rules to ban junk food sale in schools: HC. 2012, January 12). *The Times of India.* Retrieved from http://articles.timesofindia.indiatimes.com

French, C. (2009, July 11). Protective custody for 218-lb boy? *The Seattle Times.* Retrieved from http://seattletimes.nwsource.com

Fresco Menu Nutritional Brochure. (2009). *Taco Bell Corp.*

Frost, C. (2002, April). Jose Bove profile. *BBC Four.* Retrieved from http://www.bbc.co.uk/bbcfour/documentaries/profile/jose_bove.shtml

Frumkin, P. (2008, September). Menu-labeling bill headed for U.S. Senate. *Nation's Restaurant News.* Retrieved from http://www.nrn.com/article.aspx?coll_id=&keyword=menu%2011labeling&id=358730

Galea, L. (2011, March 20). *Lottery winner goes back to work at McDonald's.* [Web log post]. Retrieved from http://www.letit-flow.com/lottery-winner-goes-back-to-work-at- mcdonalds/

Gardner, A. (2011, June). Doctors urge ban on junk food ads during kids' shows. *HealthDay.* Retrieved from http://health.usnews.com/health-news/diet- fitness/diet/articles/2011/06/27/doctors-urge-ban-on-junk-food-ads-during-kids-shows

Gardner, A. (2011, November 12). Soda bans don't keep kids from sugary drinks. *USA Today.* Retrieved from http://yourlife.usato-day.com/

Gardner, D. (2011, October 21). 'A taste worth dying for': Heart Attack Grill in Las Vegas serves up 8,000 calorie burger meal… the equivalent of FIVE DAYS worth of food. *Daily Mail Online.* Retrieved from http://www.dailymail.co.uk/news/

Gay, M. (2011, April). Chicago school bans bag lunches to get kids to eat less junk food. *Aol news.* Retrieved from http://www.aol-news.com

Gengler, C. (2005). Teens and work. *University of Minnesota Extension*. Retrieved from http://www.extension.umn.edu/info-u/families/BE952.html

Giannotto, M. (2008, July 31). Fast food ban gains support among city lawmakers. *The New York Sun*. Retrieved from http://www.nysun.com/

Gibson, R. (2008, May 11). McDonald's seeks to change meaning of 'McJob.' *Press Democrat*. Retrieved from http://1.pressdemocrat.com

Givhan, R. (2010, February 10). First lady Michelle Obama: 'Let's move' and work on childhood obesity problem. *The Washington Post*. Retrieved from http://www.washingtonpost.com/wp-dyn/content/article/2010/02/09/AR2010020900791.html

Glanz, K, et al. (2007). How major restaurants plan their menus: Tthe role of profit, demand, and health [Abstract]. *Am J Prev Med*, 32(5): 383-8. Abstract retrieved from http://www.ncbi.nlm.nih.gov/pubmed/

Glick, A. (2008, June, 20). Lose weight…by eating at McDonald's. [Web log post]. Retrieved from http://glickreport.blogs.foxbusiness.com/2008/06/20/lose-weightby-eating-at-mcdonalds/

Goff, H. (2008, January). McDonald's serves up 'diplomas.' *BBC News*. Retrieved from http://news.bbc.co.uk/1/hi/education/7209276.stm

Goldmark, A. (2011, June). Without McDonald's, America would have lost jobs in May. *Good Business*. Retrieved from http://www.good.is/post/mcdonald-s-hired-more-than-all-of- the-rest-of-the-economy-combined/

Gorgan, E. (2010, September). McDonald's death ad causes a stir. *Softpedia*. Retrieved from http://news.softpedia.com/news/McDonald's-Death-Ad-Causes-a-Stir-156795.shtml

Gorman, L. (2007). TV, fast foods and childhood obesity. *The National Bureau of Economic Research*. Retrieved from http://www.nber.org/digest/aug06/w11879.html

Goody, C. (2011, July). McDonald's commitments to offer improved nutrition choices. *Today's Dietitian*. [Electronic mailing list message].

Graham, J. (2012, May 4). Obesity fight needs ambitious campaign, health leaders say. *USA Today.* Retreived from http://www.usa-today.com/

Gray, V.B., Byrd, S.H., Cossman, J.S., Chromiak, J.A., Cheek, W., & Jackson, G. (2007). Parental attitudes toward child nutrition and weight have a limited relationship with child's weight status. *Nutrition Research*, 27, 548-558. Retrieved from www.science-direct.com

Greene, B. (2009). *The best life diet.* New York, NY: Simon & Schuster Paperbacks.

Greene, B. (2004). *The get with the program! Guide to fast food & family restaurants. New* York, NY: Simon & Schuster.

greygarious. (2009, September 25). Barbara Walters vs. Paula Deen. [Web log post]. *CHOW.* Retrieved from http://chowhound.chow.com/topics/654972

Guevara, S. (2011, April 6). Proposed new rules would require menu-labeling. [Web log post]. *Consortium of Foundation Libraries.* Retrieved from http://foundationlibraries.blogspot.com/2011/04/proposed-new-rules-would-require- menu.html

Guy, S. (2003, September 17). Oprah's trainer touting meal, healthy living for McDonald's. *Chicago Sun-Times. HighBeam Research.* Retrieved from http://www.highbeam.com/doc /1P2-1500174.html

Hamblett, M. (2005, January 26). NY court revives obesity suit against McDonald's. *New York Post.* Retrieved from http://www.judicialaccountability.org/articles/mcdonaldcasedismissed .htm

Hamblett, M. (2006, September 21). NY judge lets the burgers fly in McDonald's food fight. *Citizens for Judicial Accountability. New York Law Journal.* Retrieved from http://www.judicialaccount-ability.org/articles/mcdonaldcasedismissed.htm

Harris, P.S. (2009). *None of us is as good as all of us: How McDonald's prospers by embracing inclusion and diversity.* Hoboken, NJ: John Wiley & Sons, Inc.

Hartocollis, A. (2009, October 6). Calorie postings don't change habits, study find. *The New York Times*. Retrieved from http://nytimes.com/

Hatch, A. (2010, August). Are parents of obese kids abusive? *ParentDish*. Retrieved from http://www.parentdish.com/2010/08/23/are-parents-of-obese-kids-abusive/

HBO Documentary Films., The Institute of Medicine., Centers for Disease Control and Prevention, National Institutes of Health., Michael & Susan Dell Foundation., & Kaiser Permanente. (2012). *The Weight of the Nation*. United States: HBO.

Health Day News Staff. (2011, July). Only 15% use calorie info at NYC fast food chains. *Everyday Health*. Retrieved from http://www.everydayhealth.com/diet-nutrition/0727/only-15-percent-use-calorie-info-at-nyc-fast-food-chains.aspx

Healy, M. (2011, July 7). America just keeps getting fatter. *Los Angeles Times*. Retrieved from http://www.latimes.com/

Heisler, T. (2011, July). Coming soon to your local fast food joint: alcohol? *WalletPop*. Retrieved from http://www.walletpot.com

HealthDay. (2011, August 28). Study: half of U.S. adults will be obese by 2030. *USA Today*. Retrieved from http://yourlife.usatoday.com/

Healthy Americans. (2011). *Adult obesity rates and childhood obesity rates*. Retrieved from http://healthyamericans.org/report/88/

Hellmich, N. (2011, May 5). Study: few Americans accurately monitor calories. *USA Today*. Retrieved from http://yourlife.usatoday.com/

Hellmich, N. (2011, July 13). 15,000 restaurants order healthy new kids meals. *USA Today*. http://yourlife.usatoday.com/

Hellmich, N. (2011, August 31). Sugary drinks add 300 calories a day to youths' diets. *USA Today*. Retrieved from http://yourlife.usatoday.com/

Hellmich, N. (2012, May 3). Obesity could affect 42% of Americans by 2030. *USA Today*. Retrieved from http://www.usatoday.com/

Hellmich, N. (2012, June 5). Disney to quit taking ads for junk food aimed at kids. *USA Today*. Retrieved from http://usatoday.com/

Hellmich, N. (2012, June 8). Health advocates go sour on sugar. *USA Today.* Retrieved from http://www.usatoday.com/news/health/story/2012-06-08/sugar-wars-bloomberg/55470574/1

Hernandez, D. (2011, July 17). Access to grocers doesn't improve diets, study finds. *Los Angeles Times.* Retrieved from http://articles.latimes.com/

Hess, A. (2012, January). Does banning toys make fast food healthier? *GOOD.* Retrieved from http://www.good.is/post/does-banning-toys--make-fast-food-healthier/

HighBeam Research. (1991, July.) McDonald's Corporation – McJOBS. (program for handicapped adults receives award). Article from *The Exceptional Parent.* Retrieved from http://www.highbeam.com/doc/1G1-11172284.html

Hill, M. (2010, January 8). Are those fast-food calorie counts correct? There's a fat chance they're not. *SI Live.* Retrieved from http://www.silive/com/news/index.ssf/2010/01 /are_those_fast-food_calorie_co.html

Hill, M. (2010, January 19). Restaurant calories counts sometimes off. *Mail Tribune.* Retrieved from http://www.mailtribune.com/

Hilton, P. (2009, August). *Houston's: There's a problem!* Retrieved from http://www.perezhilton.com./

Hilton, P. (2009, September). *Barbara Walters gives it to Paula Deen.* Retrieved from http://www.perezhilton.com/

Hilton, P. (2010, October). *The rich are spending more on fast food.* Retrieved from http://fitperez.com/2010-10-19-the-rich-are-spending-more-on-fast-food/?from=PH

Hirsch, J.M. (2009, February 17). The hidden calories of home cooking. *The Huffington Post.* Retrieved from http://www.huffingtonpost.com/2009/02/17/the-hidden-calories-of-ho_n_167542.html

Hoffer, S. (2011, April). World's fattest 4-year-old offered free treatment in Hong Kong. *Aol News.* Retrieved from http://www.aolnews.com/2011/04/16/worlds-fattest-4-year-old- offered-free-treatment-in-hong-kong/

Holt, B. (2011, June). Fried Kool-Aid balls are a hit. *New Jersey Newsroom*. Retrieved from http://www.newjerseynewsroom.com/style/fried-kool-aid-balls-are-a-hit

Honan, E. (2008, January). New York chain eateries must post calorie counts. *Reuters*. Retrieved from http://www.reuters.com/article/topNews/idUSN2255156520080123

Honan, E., Gorman, S., Johnston, C. (Ed.) & Beech. E. (Ed.). (2102, May). New York mayor seeks ban on sale of big sugary drinks. *Yahoo! News*. Retrieved from http://news.yahoo.com/york-mayor-bloomberg-propose-ban-sale-large-sugary-035357237–sector.html

Hook, D-L. B. (2009, August). How portion size adds up to obesity. *Every Day Health*. Retrieved from http://www.everydayhealth.com/diet-nutrition/weight-management/big-food-are-we-eating-more.aspx

Horovitz, B. (2006, April 17). McDonald's Asian-themed salad going nationwide. *USA Today*. Retrieved from http://www.usatoday.com/

Horovitz, B. (2011, July 1). Fast-food chains selling booze with burgers. *USA Today*. Retrieved from http://www.usatoday.com/

Horovitz, B. (2011, July 1). Sonic, Burger King, and other fast-food chains selling alcohol. Retrieved from http://www.usatoday.com/

Horovitz, B. (2011, November 21). Marketers adapt menus to eat-what-I-want-when-I-want trend. *USA Today*. Retrieved from http://www.usatoday.com/

Horovitz, B. (2012, February 20). Taco Bell comes out of its shell to ring in a new menu. *USA Today*. Retrieved from http://www.usatoday.com/

Horovitz, B. (2012, March 7). Chocolate milk makers now target grown-up athletes. *USA Today*. Retrieved from http://www.usatoday.com

Horovitz, B. (2012, May 11). 7-Eleven adds low-calorie Slurpee version nationwide. *USA Today*. Retrieved from http://www.usatoday.com/

Horovitz, B. (2012, May 16). Study: 96% of restaurant entrees exceed USDA limits. *USA Today.* Retrieved from http://www. usatoday.com/

Horovitz, B. (2012, May 21). Drive-throughs drive up profits for more companies. *USA Today.* Retrieved from http://www.usatoday.com/

Horovitz, B. (2012, May 31). Subway snares first seal of approval from heart group. *USA Today.* Retrieved from http://www.usatoday.com/

Horovitz, B. (2012, June 7). Coke says obesity grew as sugary drink consumption fell. *USA Today.* Retrieved from http://www.usatoday.com/

Horovitz, B. (2012, July 26). McDonald's talks up good nutrition at London games. *USA Today.* Retrieved from http://www.usatoday.com/

Hoyland, C. (Ed.). (2009, August 14). Albany County, N.Y., passes menu labeling. *QRS Web.* Retrieved from http://www.qsrweb.com/article.php?id=15508

Hsu, T. (2011, September 3). Sodium us up 144% in restaurants – mostly through gourmet salt. *Los Angeles Times.* http://latimesblogs.latimes.com/

Hsu, T. (2012, March 1). Beverly Hills Sprinkles to open 24-hour cupcake vending machine. *Los Angeles Times.* Retrieved from http://articles.latimes.com/2012/mar/01/business/la-fi- mo-sprinkles-cupcake-vending-machine-20120301

Hubbard, A. (2012, January). USDA school lunch rules 'best ever' – though pizza is still a 'vegetable.' [Web log post]. *Los Angeles Times.* Retrieved from   http://latimesblogs.latimes.com/

Hughes, K.L. (n.d.). Employment: Reasons students work. *Answers. com.* Retrieved October 18, 2008 from http://www.answers.com/topic/employment-reasons-students-work

Hui, S. (2012, June). Biggest Mac: McDonald's at Olympics is the biggest. *Yahoo! News.* Retrieved from http://news.yahoo.com/biggest-mac-mcdonalds-olympics-biggest- 165235212—oly.html

Hungry for work? What about all our wasted talent...(2012, February). *Osney Media*. Retrieved from http://osneyhr.com/ hungry-for-work-what-about-all-our-wasted-talent/

Husten, L. (Contributor). (2012, June). Subway meals get American Heart Association endorsement. *Forbes*. Retrieved from http:// www.forbes.com/sites/larryhusten/2012/06/04/ subway-meals-get-american-heart-association-endorsement/

Hutchison, C. (2011, March). Hefty Heart Attack Grill spokesman dies at 29. *ABC News*. Retrieved from http://abcnews.go.com/Health/ HeartHealth/blair-river-hefty-heart-attack-grill-spokesman-dies/ story?id=13056400

In the last 60 days, how often have you eaten at fine dining restaurants? (n.d.). *QSR Magazine*. Retrieved from http://www.qsr-magazine.com/articles/features/116/consumer_charts/8.3

In the last 60 days, how often have you eaten at fast food restaurants? (n.d.). *QSR Magazine*. Retrieved from http://www.qsrmagazine. com/articles/features/116/consumer_charts/8.1

Inman, B. (2007, March 13). For US teens unemployment levels rival those of the great depression [Web log post]. *Workforce Vision*. Retrieved from http://workforcevision.blogspot.com/2007/03/ for-us-teens-unemployment-levels-rival.html

Jacobson. M.F., Hurley, J.G. & Center for Science in the Public Interest. (2002). *Restaurant Confidential*. New York, NY: Workman Publishing Company, Inc.

Jakle, J.A., & Sculle, K.A. (1999). *Fast Food, Roadside Restaurants in the Automobile Age*. Baltimore, MD: The Johns Hopkins University Press.

Jalonick, M.C. (2011, April 27). Gov't seeks to limit junk food ads to kids. *Aol News + Huff Post*. Retrieved from http://www.aol-news.com

Jalonick, M.C. (2011, November). Pizza is a vegetable? Congress says yes. *MSNBC*. Retrieved from http://www.msnbc. msn.com/id/45306416/ns/health-diet_and_nutrition/t/ pizza-vegetable- congress-says-yes/j

Jason, (Sr. Producer). (2009, November). Michelle Obama spotlights child obesity epidemic. *Diets in Review.com* Retrieved from http://www.dietsinreview.com/diet_column/11/michelle-obama-spotlights-child-obesity-epidemic/

Jeffers, L. (with) Mayanobe, J-P. (2001). A world struggle is underway. *Z Magazine. Third World Traveler.* Retrieved from http://www.thirdworldtraveler.com/Reforming_System_/World_Struggle_Underway.html

Jennings, L. (2007, September). California pols pass statewide menu-labeling requirements. *Nations Restaurant News.* Retrieved from http://findarticles.com/p/articles/mi_m3190/is_/ai_n27391262

JLP. (2008, July). L.A. wants a year-long ban on fast food. Retrieved from http://allfinancialmatters.com/2008/07/29/la-wants-a-year-long-ban-on-fast-food/

Johnson, W.B. (2011, March 3). 575-ound Heart Attack Grill spokesman dies. *The Arizona Republic.* Retrieved from http://www.azcentral.com/

Jones, D.J. (Ed.). (2008). *Nutrition in the fast lane: A guide to nutrition and dietary exchange values for fast food.* Indianapolis, IN: Franklin Publishing Incorporated.

jorge. (2010, July 7). 10 largest fast food chains in the U.S. by location. [Web log post].

EZlocal Blog. Retrieved from http://ezlocal.com/blog/post/10-Largest-Fast-Food-Chains_in-the-US.aspx

Jose Bove – the man who dismantled a McDonald's. (2004, April). *H2g2.* Retrieved from http://www.h2g2.com/approved_entry/A706736.

Joseph, S. (2010). *Ban trans fats: The campaign to ban partially hydrogenated oils.* Retrieved from http://www.bantransfats.com/

Judge nixes lawsuit against McDonald's. (2003, September). *redOrbit.* Retrieved from http://www.redorbit.com

Kahn, A. (2006, January 10). Gaining weight? Maybe you should blame nutrition labels. [Web log post]. *Los Angeles Times.* Retrieved from http://latimesblogs.latimes.com/

Kaiser Pemanente. (2000). *A guide for my diabetes care.* Woodland Hills, CA: Regional Health Education.

Kaiser Permanente. (2003). *Eat hearty cholesterol class.* Woodland Hills, CA: Health Education.

Kaiser Permanente. (2003). *Healthy eating for adults.* Woodland Hills, CA: Health Education.

Kaiser Permanente. (2006). *Fast food: A guide to healthier choices.* SCPMG: Regional Health Education.

Kaiser Permanente. (2000-2009). *Cultivating health weight management kit.* Health Education Services.

Kane, C. (2012, July). America's weirdest restaurants. *Yahoo! Finance.* Retrieved from http://finance.yahoo.com/news/america-s-weirdest-restaurants.html

Keaton, J. (2001, August). French farmer Jose Bove leads new McDonald's protest. *Associated Press.* Retrieved from http://www.commondreams.org/headlines01/0813-01.htm

Kessler, D.A. (2009). *The end of overeating. Taking control of the insatiable American appetite.* New York, NY: Rodale.

Kids fare at sit-down restaurants is often worse than fast food. (n.d.). *iHealthtube.* Retrieved from http://www.ihealthtube.com/aspx/article.aspx?id=147

KFC. (2008). *About us.* Retrieved from http://www.kfc.com/about/

KFC. (2012). *Nutrition.* Retrieved from http://www.kfc.com/nutrition/

Kincheloe, J.L. (2002). *The sign of the burger, McDonald's and the culture of power.* Philadelphia, PA: Temple University Press.

Kingson, J. A. (1988, March 6). Ideas & trends; golden years spent under golden arches. *The New York Times.* Retrieved from http://query.nytimes.com

Kinsley, M. (2002, July). A lawsuit to choke on. *TIME. CNN.* Retrieved from http://www.time.com/time/printout/0,8816,332981,00.html

Kish, M. (2006, February 27). Banning 'Mclawsuits'; state bill outlawing fast-food litigation nears passage. *Small Biz.*

Retrieved from http://www.judicialaccountability.org/articles/mcdonaldcasedismissed.htm

Kluger, J. (2010, January). Study: calorie counts often wrong on food labels. *TIME*. Retrieved from http://www.time.com/time/health/article/0,8599,1951798,00.html

Knowledge@Wharton. (2007, May). *Serving up smaller restaurant portions: Will consumers Bite?* Retrieved from http://knowledge.wharton.upenn.edu/article.cfm?articleid=1737

Knowles, D. (2010, March). Weight Watchers will promote McDonald's menu items in New Zealand. *AoL News*. Retrieved from http://www.aolnews.com/2010/03/04/weight-watchers-you-deserve-a-break-at-mcdonalds/

Kramer, N. (1995, April). Employee benefits for older workers. *Monthly Labor Review*. Retrieved from http://findarticles.com/p/articles/mi_m1153/is_n4_v118/ai_16898387/pg_6

Krieger, E. (2012, March 20). Is oversnacking becoming the norm in our nation? *USA Today*. Retrieved from http://www.usatoday.com/

LA may ban new fast-food restaurants. (2008, July). *KNBC*. Retrieved from http://www.knbc.com/news/16959136/detail.html

Lane, R.M., & McCorkle, M. (2003). Employment & volunteer opportunities for seniors. *Alabama Cooperative Extension System*. Retrieved from http://www.aces.edu/pubs/docs/U/UNP-0005/

Lang, S. (2009, February). 'Joy of Cooking' supersizes and packs more calories into home cooking. *Cornell University Chronicle Online*. Retrieved from http://www.news.cornell.edu/stories/Feb09/JoyCookingPortions.html

Lehman, J. (2003, September 5). Judge purges fatties' Mcsuit. *New York Post*. Retrieved from http://www.judicialaccountability.org/articles/mcdonaldcasedismissed.htm

Lempert, P. (2011, March 7). *Healthy eating: home vs. restaurants.* [Web log post]. Retrieved from http://www.philsfoodsense.org/2011/03/07/1030/

Lentini, N.M. (2007, April 16). Riding sales wave, McDonald's intros new premium salad. *Media Post News*. Retrieved from http://www.mediapost.com

Leshock, M. (n.d.). Fried Kool-Aid?! 16 ridiculous fried fair foods. *WGNTV*. Retrieved from http://www.wgntv.com/blogs/leshock-value/wgntv-fried-koolaid-16-ridiculous-fried-fair- foods-photos-20110620,0,5336253.photogallery

Leung, R. (2007, December). The Subway diet. *CBS News*. Retrieved from http://www.cbsnews.com/2100-18559_162-603484.html

Lin, Joanna. (n.d.). Menus list calories, but Californians may not be counting. *California Watch*. Retrieved from http://california-watch.org

Loeb, M. (2008, May). The longer you work the longer – and better – your life. *Yahoo! Finance*. Retrieved from http://finance.yahoo.com

Los Angeles fast-food restaurant ban unlikely to have impact on obesity. (2009, October). *RAND*. Retrieved from http://www.rand.org/news/press/2009/10/06.html

Love, D. (2011, April). 15 successful people who started their careers at McDonald's. *Business Insider*. Retrieved from http://www.businessinsider.com/celebrities-who-used-to-work-at- mcdonalds?op=1

Love, J.F. (1995). *McDonald's: Behind the arches*. New York, NY: Bantam Books.

Lubin, G. (2012, April 30). 13 disturbing facts about McDonald's. *The Fiscal Times*. Retrieved from http://www.thefiscaltimes.com/

Lynch, R. (2011, November 7). As income rises, so does fast-food consumption, study finds. [Web log post]. *Los Angeles Times*. Retrieved from http://latimesblogs.latimes.com/

MacDougall, W. (2003). Shaking the golden arches. *CounterPunch*. Retrieved from http://www.counterpunch.org/macdougall01092003.html

Macaroni Grill. (2012). *Nutrition information*. Retrieved from http://www.macaronigrill.com/docs/nutritional/nutritional-menu.pdf

Mackey, M. (2012, April 25). Dying for a burger? Try the Heart Attack Grill. *The Fiscal Times*. Retrieved from http://www.the-fiscaltimes.com/

Mahan, K., & Escott-Stump, S. (2004). *Krause's food, nutrition & diet therapy* (11th ed). Philadelphia: Saunders.

Malcolm, H. (2012, January 30). Devices let you check calories in snack machines. *USA Today*. Retrieved from http://www.usato-day.com

Marchetta, T. (2010, May 4). Are menu calorie counts accurate? *Denver News*. Retrieved from http://www.thedenverchannel.com/news/23422590/detail.html

Marketwire. (2010). *McDonald's new fundraising efforts bring families together, showing how small donations can add up to make a big difference.* Retrieved from http://www.marketwire.com/press-release/McDonalds-New-Fundraising-Efforts-Bring-Families-Together-Showing-How-Small-Donations-1296778.htm

Martin, R. (1984, February). Training of handicapped garners national plaudits – in fast food industry. *Nation's Restaurant News*. Retrieved from http://findarticles.com/p/articles/mi_m 3190/is_/ai/3136667

McDonald's targeted in obesity lawsuit. (2002, November). *BBC News*. Retrieved from http://news.bbc.co.uk/2/hi/americas/2502431.stm

McDonalds once again tops list of best companies for minorities. (2004, July). *QSR Web*. Retrieved from http://www.qsr.web.com/article.php?id=419

McDonald's to hire 50,000 workers – in 1 day. (2011, April). *CNN Money*. Retrieved from http://money.cnn.com/2011/04/04/news/companies/mcdonalds_jobs/index.htm

McDonald's. (2012). *Nutrition*. Retrieved from www.mcdonalds.com/us/en/food/food/nutrition_choices.html

McDonald's 2012 Olympic plans include its largest unit in the world. (n.d.). *QSR Web*. Retrieved from http://www.qsrweb.com/article_print/182671/McDonald-s-2012-Olympic-plans-include-its-largest-unit-in-the-world

McDonald's Corporation. (2006a). *Bob Greene*. Retrieved from http://www.mcdonald's.com/us/en/home.html

McDonald's Corporation. (2006b). *McDonald's recognized as a partner in the community*. Retrieved from http://www.mcdonalds.com/

McDonald's Corporation. (2006c). *McDonald's commitment to communites*. Retrieved from http://www.mcdonalds.com/

McDonald's Corporation. (2006d). *McDonald's is a local business that invests in local communities*. Retrieved from http://www.mcdonalds.com/

McDonald's Corporation. (2006e). *Fact sheet Ronald McDonald House Charites*. Retrieved from http://www.mcdonalds.com/

McDonald's Corporation. (2006f). *McDonald's Facts Summary*. Retrieved from http://www.mcdonalds.com/

McDonald's raises millions for world children's day. (2007, November). *QSR Magazine*. Retrieved from http://www.qsr-magazine.com/articles/news/story.phtml?id=5871

McDonald's Corporation. (2008a). *Commitment to Diversity*. Retrieved from http://www. Mcdonalds.com/

McDonald's Corporation. (2008b). *Employer awards and recognition*. Retrieved from http://www.mcdonalds.com/corp/career/awards_recognition.html

McDonald's Corporation. (2008c). *Hamburger university*. Retrieved from http://www.mcdonalds.com/corp/career/hamburger_university.html

McDonald's Corporation. (2008d). *About McDonald's...* Retrieved from http://www.mcdonalds.com/corp/about.html

McDonald's Corporation. (2008e). *Community giving*. Retrieved from http://www.mcdonalds.com/corp/values/place/community_giving.html

McDonald's Corporation. (2008f). *McDonald's corporate careers*. Retrieved from http://www.mcdonalds.com/corp/career.html.

McDonald's Corporation. (2008g). *Ralph Alvarez, president and chief operating officer*. Retrieved from http://www.aboutmcdonalds.com/mcd/our_company/bios/ralph_alvarez. html

McDonald's Corporation. (2008h). *Richard Floersch, executive vice president – chief human resources officer.* Retrieved from http://www. aboutmcdonalds.com/mcd/our_company/ leadership/richard_ floersch.html

McDonald's Corporation. (2008i). *Karen King, east division president – McDonald's USA.* Retrieved from http://www.aboutmcdonalds.com/mcd/our_company/bios/karen_king.html

McDonald's Corporation. (2008j). *Gloria Santona, executive vice president, general counsel and secretary.* Retrieved from http:// www.aboutmcdonalds.com/mcd/our_comapny/bios/ gloria_ santona.html

McDonald's Corporation. (2008k*). Jeff Stratton, executive vice president and chief restaurant Officer.* Retrieved from http://www.aboutmcdonalds.com/mcd/our_company/bios/jeff_ stratton.html

McDonald's Corpoation. (2008l). *Fred L. Turner, honorary chairman.* Retrieved from http://www.aboutmcdonalds.com/mcd/ our_company/bios/fred_l_turner.html

McDonald's Corporation. (2008m). *McDonald's USA food exchanges.* Retrieved from http://nutrition.mcdonalds.com/bagamcmeal/ nutrition_exchanges.hmtl

McDonald's Corporation. (2008n). *The McDonald's history – 1954 to 1955.* Retrieved from http://www.mcdonalds.com/corp/about/ mcd_history_pg1.html

McDonald's Corporation (2008o). *Diversity and employment.* Retrieved from http://www.mcdonalds.com/corp/values/people/diversity/employment.html

McDonald's Corporation. (2009a). *Jose Armario, group president – McDonald's Canada and Latin America.* Retrieved from http:// www.aboutmcdonalds.com/mcd/our_company/bios/jose-armario.html

McDonald's Corporation. (2009b). *Tim Fenton, president – Asia, Pacific, Middle East and Africa.* Retrieved from http://www. aboutmcdonalds.com/mcd/our_comapny/bios/tim_fenton. html

McDonald's Corporation. (2009c). *Janice L. Fields, executive vice president and chief operating officer – McDonald's USA.* Retrieved from http://www.aboutmcdonalds.com/mcd/our_company/bios/Janice_l_fields.html

McDonald's Corporation. (2009d). *Denis Hennequin, president – McDonald's Europe.* Retrieved from http://www.aboutmcdonalds.com/mcd/our_company/bios/denis_hennequin.html

McDonald's Corporation. (2009e). *Steve Plotkin, west division president – McDonald's USA.* Retrieved from http://www.aboutmcdonalds.com/mcd/our_company/bios/steve_plotkin.html

McDonald's Corporation. (2009f). *Jim Skinner, vice chairman and chief executive officer.* Retrieved from http://www.aboutmcdonalds.com/mcd/our_company/bios/jim_skinner.html

McDonald's Corporation. (2009g). *Don Thompson, president McDonald's USA.* Retrieved from http://www.aboutmcdonalds.com/mcd/our_company/bios/don_thompson.html

McDonald's Corporation. (2009h). *McDonald's #1 in Fortune's most admired food services companies list.* Retrieved from http://www.crmcdonalds.com

McDonald's Corporation. (2011a). *Response to WSJ health care article.* Retrieved from http://www.aboutmcdonalds.com/mcd/newsroom/mcdonalds_statements_and_alerts/response_to_WSJ_healthcare_article.html

McDonald's Corporation. (2011b). *Opportunity at McDonald's.* Retrieved from http://www.aboutmcdonalds.com/

McDonald's Corporation. (2011c). *Diversity at McDonald's.* Retrieved from http://http://www.aboutmcdonalds.com/content/mcd/students/serving_our_communities/diversity.html

McDonald's Corporation. (2011d). *Corporate accolades.* Retrieved from http://www.aboutmcdonalds.com/mcd/our_company/corporate_accolades.html

McDonald's Corporation. (2011, April). We Believe. *Us Weekly.*

McDonald's tops Fortune Mag's minority survey. (2004, July). *QSR Magazine.* Retrieved from http://www.qsrmagazine.com/articles/news/story.phtml?id=4269

References

McDonald's seeks all-American achievers. (2008, October). *QSR Magazine.* Retrieved from http://www.qsrmagazine.com/articles/news/story.phtml?id=7403

McDonald's USA. (2008). *McDonald's nutrition facts.* Retrieved from http://nutrition.mcdonalds.com/bacamcmeal/nutrition facts.html

McDonald's welcomes parents to work. (2008, October). *QSR Magazine.* Retrieved from http://www.qsrmagazine.com/articles/news/story.phtml?id=6442

Mcjob. (2008). *Merriam-Webster.* Retrieved from http://mw1.m-w.com/dictionary/mcjob

McJobs program cited for aiding mentally retarded. (1991, July). Retrieved from http://findarticles.com/p/ariticles/mi_m3190/is_n28_v25/ai_10996841.

McKenzie, J. (January). Food portion sizes have grown – a lot. *ABC News.* Retrieved from http://abcnews.go.com/WNT/story?id=129685&page=1

McSpotlight. (2008, November). *The issues.* Retrieved from http://www.mcspotlight.org/ issues/intro.html

Media and childhood obesity. (n.d.). *Parent's Place.* Retrieved from http://reboot.fcc.gov/parents/media-and-childhood-obesity

Medina, J. (2011, January). In South Los Angeles, new fast-food spots get a 'no, thanks.' *The New York Times.* Retrieved from http://www.nytimes.com/

Medina, J. (2011, December 18). Fast-food outlet stirs concern in a mecca of healthy living. *The New York Times.* Retrieved from http://www.nytimes.com

Mercola, J. (2002). [Peer commentary on *U.S. junk food intake worsening.* Presented at the Annual Experimental Biology 2002 Conference in New Orleans, LA]. Retrieved from http://articles.mercola.com/sites/articles/archive/2002/05/08/junk-food-part-one.aspx

Mercola, J. (2003) [Peer commentary on *Food portions increase along with obesity. JAMA 289: 450-453.* Retrieved from http://articles.

mercola.com/sites/articles/archive/2003/02/05 food-portions.
aspx

Michaelson, E. (2010, December). S. LA bans new stand-alone fast
food eateries. *KABC-TV.* Retrieved from http://abclocal.go.com/
kabc/story?section=news/local/los_angeles&id =7831475

Miller, D. (2008, June). Ban on fast food proposed for South Los
Angeles; councilwoman wants McDonald's, KFC, off menu. *Los
Angeles Business Journal.* Retrieved from http://www.allbusiness.
com/legal/trial-procedure-ordinances/11471475-1.html

Miller, T. (2009, July 22). Is child obesity abuse? Court to decide if
S.C. mom Jerry Gray neglected 555-pound, 14-year-old son.
NY Daily News. Retrieved from http://articles.nydailynews.com

Modugno, B. (2009, July). From McDonald's SoCal nutritionists.
[Web log post]. *McDonald's Southern California.* Retrieved
from http://www.mcdonaldssocal.com/nutritionists-blog

Mohajer, S.T. (2011, September). FDA cooking up helpful new
nutrition facts label. *Yahoo! News.* Retrieved from http://
news.yahoo.com/fda-cooking-helpful-nutrition-facts-label-
203605860.html

Moore, R. (2009, August). The real 'Julie' not as nice as Amy, 'Julie
& Julia' blogger admits. *Orlando Sentinel.* Retrieved from http://
www.orlandosentinel.com/entertainment/orl-story- julie-pow-
ell-interview,0,380028.storybvvvvn

Morantz, A. (2001, Quarter 2). Teens in the workforce. *Regional
Review.* Retrieved from http://www.bos.frb.org/economic/nerr/
rr2001q2/teens/htm

More Americans enjoying an evening out. (2011, July). *Marist
Poll.* Retrieved from http://maristpoll.marist.edu/720-more
-americans-enjoying-an-evening-out/

morganwrites. (2008, August). *South L.A. and the new fast-food ban.*
Retrieved from http://morganwrites.wordpress.com/2008/08/
23/south-la-and-the-news-fast-food-ban/

Murphy, E. (2011, November). Fast food's biggest fans aren't who
you'd think. *Daily Finance.* Retrieved from http://www.daily-

finance.com/2011/11/09/fast-foods-biggest-fans-arent-who
-youd-think/

Myrdal, A. (2002). *American kids' poor food choices: Fewer than 15
percent eat recommended fruits and vegetables.* Retrieved April 16,
2008 from http://www.eurekaalert.org/pub_releases/2002-05/
pn-akp051602.php

Nader, C. (2007, February). $330,000 buys maccas the
tick of approval. *The Age.* Retrieved from http://www.
theage.com.au/news/national/330000-buys-tick-of-appro
val/2007/02/05/1170524026024.html

Nader, A. (2012, March 7). Sprinkles cupcakes vending machines to
hit Manhattan. *The Village Voice.* Retrieved from http://blogs.vil-
lagevoice.com/forkintheroad/2012/ 03/cupcake_vending.php

Nash/Helsinki, J.M. (2003, August). Obesity goes global. *TIME
Magazine.* Retrieved from http://www.time.com/time/maga-
zine/article/0,9171,1101030825-476417,00.html

Nation's Restaurant News. (2005, April). *Diversity at McDonald's:
A way of life.* Retrieved from http://findarticles.com/p/articles/
mi_m3190/is_15_39/ai_n13649047

National Center for Chronic Disease Prevention and Health
Promotion Division of Nutrition Physical Activity, and Obesity.
(n.d.). *Incorporating away-from-home food into a healthy eating
plan.* Research to Practice Series, No. 6.

National Institutes of Health. (2005). *Decline in physical activity
plays key role in weight gain among adolescent girls.* Retrieved from
http://www.nih.gov/news/pr/jul2005/nhlbi-13.htm

National Institute on Media and the Family. (2006). *Media use and
obesity among children.* Retrieved from http://www.mediafamily.
org/facts/facts_tvandobchild.shtml

National Restaurant Association. (2009). *Public policy issue briefs:
Menu labeling/nutrition information.* Retrieved from http://www.
restaurant.org/government/Issues/Issu.cfm?Issue= Menulabel

National Restaurant Association. (2011). *National restaurant association's first-of-its-kind "Kids LiveWell"initiative showcases restau-*

rants' healthful menu options for children. Retrieved from http://www.restaurant.org/pressroom/pressrelease/?ID=2136

National Science Foundation. (2005). *2003 college graduates in the U.S. workforce: a profile.* Retrieved from http://www.nsf.gov/statistics/infbrief/nsf06304/

Nearly 48,000 diners rate best & worst at 102 popular restaurant chains. (2012, June). *Consumer Reports.* Retrieved from http://pressroom.consumerreports.org/pressroom/2012/06/my-entry- 6.html

Neergard, L. (n.d.). Brain cues may lead to overeating. *The Daily News.*

Nelson, N. (2010, May 19). At Burgerville, get a burger, fries and a guilt trip. [Web log post]. *Slashfood.* Retrieved from http://www.slashfood.com/2010/05/19/at-burgerville-order-up-a- burger-fries-and-a-guilt-trip/

Nemours Foundation. (2007). *Even the youngest kids watch TV daily.* Reviewed by Dowshen, S., MD. Retrieved from http://kidshealth.org/research/tv_kids.html

Nemours Foundation. (2008). *How TV affects your child.* Reviewed by Gavin, M.L., MD. Retrieved from http://kidshealth.org/parent/positive/family/tv_affects_child.html

Nestle, M. (2002, 2007). *Food politics.* Berkley and Los Angeles, CA: University of California Press.

Neumark-Sztainer, D., Story, M., Hannan, P.J., & Croll, J. (2002). Overweight status and eating patterns among adolescents: Where do youths stand in comparison with the Healthy People 2010 objectives? *Am J Public Health*, 92(5), 844-851. Retrieved from http://www.pubmedcentral.nih.gov/articlerender.fcgi?artid=1447172

New York City Department of Health and Mental Hygiene. (2010). *Cardiovascular disease prevention.* Retrieved from http://www.nyc.gov/html/doh/html/cardio/cario-transfat.shtml

New York City passes trans fat ban: Restaurants must eliminate artery-clogging ingredient by July 2008. (2006, December 5). *Msnbc.*Retrieved from http://www.msnbc.com/id/ 16051436/

Newman, J. (2007). *My secret life on the McJob: Lessons from behind the counter guaranteed to supersize any management style.* New York, NY: McGraw-Hill.

Nichols, M. (2011, April 5). New York City to consider banning fast-food toys. *Reuters.* Retrieved from http://www.reuters.com/

NIDDK. (2007). *Statistics related to overweight and obesity.* Retrieved April 13, 2008 from http://win.niddk.nig.gov/statistics/index.htm

Nielsen, J., Siega-Riz, A.M., & Popkin, B.M. (2002). Trends in energy intake in U.S. between 1977 and 1996: Similar shifts seen across age groups. *Obes Res.*10, 370-378.

Northcutt, W. (2003). Jose Bove vs. McDonald's: The making of a national hero in the French anti-globalization movement. *Niagra University.* Retrieved from http://quod.lib.umich.edu/w/wsfh/0642292.0031.020?rgn=main;view=fulltext

NRA, healthy dining launch healthy menu initiative for kids. (n.d.). *QSR Web.* Retrieved from http://www.qsrweb.com/article_print/182533/NRA-Healthy-Dining-launch-healthy-menu- initiative-for-kids

NY Metro McDonald's. (2009). *McDonald's New York Tri-State area restaurants celebrate take your parent to work month.* Retrieved from http://www.mcdonaldsnymetro.com /en/291/take-your-parents-to-work-month-4-23-09

NY orders calories posted on chain menus. (2008, January). *CNN Health.* Retrieved from http://articles.cnn.com/2008-01-22/health/calories.menus_1_calorie-counts-calorie-information-menus?_s=PM:HEALTH

Obese children show signs of heart disease typically seen in middle-aged adults, researcher says. (2010, October). *Science Daily.* Retrieved from http://www.sciencedaily.com/releases/2010/10/101025005834.htm#.UEgJqqOi-pw.emailhttp://www.sciencedaily.com/releases/2010/10/101025005834.htm#.UEgJqqOi- pw.email

Obesity begins at home – segment two. [Television broadcast]. (n.d.). *Scientific American Frontiers. PBS.* Retrieved from http://www.pbs.org/saf/1110/segments/1110-2.htm

Obesity: In statistics, people are getting fatter almost everywhere in the world. (2008, January). *BBC News.* Retrieved from http://news.bbc.co.uk/2/hi/health/7151813.stm

Obesity lawsuit weighed again.(2005, January 26). *The Washington Times.* Retrieved from http://www.washingtontimes.com

Obesity rate 30% in 12 states of the US. (2011, July 20). *Medical News Today.* Retrieved from http://www.medicalnewstoday.com/articles/231423.php

O'Dougherty, M., Harnack, L.J., French, S.A., Story, M., Oakes, J.M. & Jeffrey, R.W. (2006, March-April). Menu labeling and value size pricing at fast-food restaurants: a consumer perspective. *Am J Health Promot.* 20(4), 247-50.

Ogilvie, J.P. (2011, August 29). Pro/con: Does obesity qualify as child abuse? *Los Angeles Times.* Retrieved from http://www.latimes.com/

Oldenburg, A. (2011, February 21). Rush Limbaugh attacks Michelle Obama's diet. *USA Today.* Retrieved from http://content.usatoday.com/communities/entertainment/post/2011/02/rush-limbaugh-attacks-michelle-obamas-diet/1

Oldenburg, A. (2012, January 17). Wendy Williams launches 'save the Twinkie' campaign. *USA Today.* Retrieved from http://content.usatoday.com

Olive Garden. (2012). *Nutrition.* Retrieved from http://www.olivegarden.com/Menu/Nutrition/

One-Off Productions. (1997). *George Ritzer, author of "the McDonaldization of society"* Retrieved from http://www.mcspotlight.org/people/interviews/ritzer_george.html

O'Neill, B. (2009, July). Choking on the facts. *Spiked.* Retrieved from http://www.spiked-online.com/index.php?/site/article/2477/

Orgill, J. (2011, April 10). Labeling our menus; changing our choices. [Web log post]. *Sanford Journal of Public Policy.* Retrieved from http://sjpp.duke.edu/2011/labeling -menus-changing-choices/

Ortiz, J. (2007, August 4). More restaurants adjust to rising takeout demand. *The Record Searchlight*. Retrieved from http://www.redding.com/news/

Ossad, J. (2011, April). New York City lawmaker proposes fast-food toy ban. *CNN U.S.* Retrieved from http://articles.cnn.com

Outback Steakhouse. (n.d.). *Nutrition*. Retrieved from http://www.outback.com/menu/nutritionselection.aspx?gclid=CJ6jvJ- BorICFQSxnQodD2IA4Q

Overley, J., & Koerner, C. (2010, July 15). Deep-fried and oversized at 2010 OC fair. *The Orange County Register*. Retrieved from http://foodfrenzy.ocregister.com/

Paddock, R.C. (2010, April). California county bans toys with fast-food meals. *Aol News*. http://www.aolnews.com/

Paeratakul, S., Ferdinand, D.P., Champagne, C.M., Ryan, D.H., & Bray, G.A. Fast-food consumption among US adults and children: dietary and nutrient intake profile. (2003). *J Am Diet Assoc*. 103(10): 1332-8. Retrieved from http://www.ncbi.nlm.nih.gov/

Palo Alto Medical Foundation. (n.d). *Fast food*. Retrieved from http://www.pamf.org/teen /health/nutrition/fastfood.html

Parento, E. W. (2009, February). Menu labeling laws – sweeping the nation? [Web log post]. Retrieved from http://firstmovers.blogspot.com/2009/02/menu-labeling-laws-sweeping-nation 22.html

Park, M. (2010, August 5). About 60 percent pay attention to nutrition facts. [Web log post]. *The Chart – CNN.com*. Retrieved from http://thechart.blogs.cnn.com/2010/08/05/about- 60-percent-pay-attention-to-nutrition-facts/

Parseghian, P. (2009, June). Operators, experts say calories count little in the eyes of guests. *Nation's Restaurant News*. Retrieved from http://www.nrn.com/article/operators-experts-say -calories-count-little -eyes-guests

Patrecca, L. (2012, July 9). Coke, Pepsi and others launch assault against NYC soda ban. *USA Today*. Retrieved from http://www.usatoday.com/

Patton, L. (2011, April). McDonald's hires 62,000 in U.S. event, 24% more than planned. *Bloomberg.* Retrieved from http://www.bloomberg.com/news/2011-04-28/mcdonald-s-hires-62-000-during-national-event-24-more-than-planned.html

Payne, W.T. (2008). The surprising number of Americans who have actually worked at McDonald's. *Helium.* Retrieved from http://www.helium.com

PayScale. (2008). *Salary survey report for job: Waiter/waitress.* Retrieved from http://www.payscale.com/research/US/Job=Waiter%2FWaitress/Salary

PayScale. (2008). *Hourly rate survey report for job: Sales clerk/cashier.* Retrieved from http://www.payscale.com/research/US/Job=Sales_Clerk%2FCashier/Hourly_Rate

PayScale. (2008). *Hourly rate survey report for industry: Retail grocery.* Retrieved from http://www.payscale.com/research/US/Industry=Retail_Grocery/Hourly_Rate

PayScale. (2008). *Median hourly rate by years experience for job: Stock clerk, grocery Store (United States).* Retrieved from http://www.payscale.com/research/US/Job=Stock_ Clerk_Grocery_Store/Hourly_Rate

PBS – Scientific American Frontiers. (2001). *Fat and happy?: Obesity begins at home.* [Synopsis television series episode.]. Retrieved from http://www.pbs.org/saf/1110/segments /1110-2.htm

Pearce, J., Blakely, T., Witten, & K., Bartie, P. (2007). Neighborhood deprivation and access to fast-food retailing: A national study. *Am J Prev Med.* 32(5).

People eat more calories at 'health' restaurants, Cornell study finds. (2007). *Fox News.* Retrieved from http://www.foxnews.com/story/0,2933,300334,00.html

Pepin, J. (1998, December). Ray Kroc: McDonald's begat an industry because a 52-year-old mixer salesman understood that we don't dine – we eat and run. *TIME Magazine.* Retrieved from http://www.time.com/time/1ime100/builder/profile/kroc.html.

Percentage of obese residents by state. (2012, August 14). *USA Today.* Retrieved from http://www.usatoday.com/

Perman, S. (2009). *In-N-Out burger: A behind-the-counter look at the fast-food chain that breaks all the rules.* New York, NY: Collins Business.

PETA's bloody 'unhappy meals' making parents angry. (2009, August). *Fox News.* Retrieved from http://www.foxnews.com/story/0,2933,538821,00.html

PETA (2009). *Inside PETA'S unhappy meal.* Retrieved from http://www.mccruelty.com/ unhappyMeal.aspx

Polis, C. (2012, January 3). Fast food toy ban does improve nutritional promotion but not actual menu items, says study. *Huffington Post.* Retrieved from http://huffingtonpost.com /2012/01/03/fast-food-toy-ban_n_1181325.html

Pollen, M. (2009). *Food rules: An eater's manual.* New York, NY: Penguin Books.

Pomeranz, J. (2008, September). Response to posts regarding menu labeling. *Wellsphere.* Retrieved from http://stanford.wellsphere.com/obesity-article/response-to-posts-regarding-menu-labeling/

Portnoy, H. (2012, January 15). CA town attempts to ban McDonald's on religious grounds. *Libertarian Examiner.* Retrieved from http://www.examiner.com/libertarian-in-national/

Powell, L.M., Chaloupka, F.J., & Yanjun, B. (2007). The availability of fast-food and full- service restaurants in the United States: Associations with neighborhood characteristics. *Am J Prev Med,* 33(4S).

Powell, L.M., Szczypka, B.A., & Chaloupka, F.J. (2007). Adolescent exposure to food adverstising on television. *Am J Prev Med,* 33(4S).

Preidt, R. (2010, October). Arteries of obese kids aging prematurely: Study. *Health.* Retrieved from http://news.health.com/2010/10/25/arteries-of-obese-kids-aging-prematurely-study/

Prentice, A.M., & Jebb, S.A. (2003). Fast foods, energy density and obesity: A possible mechanistic link. *Obesity Reviews,* 4(4), 187-194. Doi:10.1046/j.1467-789X.2003. 00117.x

Presky, D. (2008, July). Ronald McDonald House helps families. *KXNet.com.* Retrieved from http://www.kxmb.com/t/halliday-nd/257430.asp

PRNewswire. (2010, July). McDonald's (R) unveils R Gym (TM): The new and fun way for kids to play. Retrieved from http://www2.prnewswire.com/cgi-bin/stories.pl?ACCT=104&STORY=/www/story/07-07-2006/0004393223&EDATE

PRNewswire. (2005, January). Article: Bob Greene renews 'go active' relationship with McDonald's(R); Oprah's personal trainer and McDonald's build on unprecedented balanced active lifestyles' commitment. *High Beam Research.* Retrieved from http://www.highbeam.com/doc/1G1-126877633.html

Public Health Seattle & King County. (2008). *Nutrition menu labeling and artificial trans fat.* Retrieved from http://www.metrokc.gov/health/healthyeating

Quaid, L. (2008, October 24). One in four U.S. students dropping out. *The Daily News.*

Quigg, B. (2009, November). Working your way up the food chain. *PayScale.* Retrieved from http://jobs.aol.com/articles/photos/fast-food-jobs-and-what-they-pay/2475551/

Rappoport, L. (2003). *How we eat.* Toronto, Ontario, Canada: ECW Press.

Raskin, H. (2010, November 12). Calorie count evasion: For a limited time only, the really good stuff. [Web log post]. *Dallas Observer.* Retrieved from http://blogs.dallasobserver.com/cityofate/2010/11/calorie_count_evasion_as_if_we.php

Red Lobster. (2012). *Nutrition facts.* Retrieved from http://www.redlobster.com/health/nutrition/dinner.asp

Rees, D. (2008). Children at risk. *Illinois Nutrition Education and Training Program.* Retrieved from http://www.kidseatwell.org/riskofchildren.html

Reheating a deep fried case. (2005, January). *CFIF.* Retrieved from http://www.cfif.org/htdocs/legal_issues/legal_updates/other_noteworthy_cases/mcdonalds-_lawsuit-htm

Reinberg, S. (2011, August). Too much TV may take years off your life. *Yahoo! News.* Retrieved from http://news.yahoo.com/too-much-tv-may-years-off-lief-231005195.html

Reingold, E.M. (2001, June). America's hamburger helper. *TIME Magazine.* Retrieved from http://www.time.com/time/magazine/article/0,9171,159962.html?iid=chix-sphere

Reinke, B.B. (n.d.). Dining out done right. *The Christian Broadcasting Network.* Retrieved from http://www.cbn.com/health/nutrition/reinke_diningout.aspx?option=print

Restaurant News. (2010, December). *Yum! Brands issues 2010 corporate responsibility report "serving the world."* Retrieved from http://www.restaurantnews.com/tag/kfc/

Rettner, R. (2011, January). Menu nutrition labels don't change habits. *MSNBC.* Retrieved from http://www.msnbc.msn.com/id/41078893/ns/health-diet_and_nutrition/t/menu-nutrition-_labels-dont-change-habits/

Reuters. (2002, March). French activist gets jail for McDonald's attack. *Common Dreams.* Retrieved from http://www.commondreams.org/headlines.shtml?/headlines02/0206-02.htm

Reuters. (2011, June). U.S. doctors: Ban fast food ads on TV. *Fox News.* Retrieved from http://www.foxnews.com/health/2011/06/27/us-doctors-ban-fast-food-ads-on-tv/

Reuters Limited. (2008, May). McDonald's fries are now trans fat-free in U.S., Canada. *USA Today.* Retrieved from http://www.usatoday.com/money/industries/food/2008-05-22-_Mcdonalds-trans-fat_.html

Reynolds, D. (2010, February). California adopts trans-fat ban. *Health.* Retrieved from http://www.emaxhealth.com/1506/74/35007/california-adopts-trans-fat-ban.html

Rice, S. (2010, May 25). Restaurants take calories to the extreme, report says. *CNN Health.* Retrieved from http://thechart.blogs.cnn.com/2010/05/25/restaurants-take-calories-to-the-_extreme-report-says/

Rindfleisch, T. (2010, April). Fast food can be healthy, McDonald's dietitian says. *Sun Sentinel.* Retrieved from http://articles.sun-sentinel.com/2010-04-27/business/ sfl-mcdonalds-nutrition- 042210_1_mcdonald-nutrition-goody

Ritzer, G. (2002). *An Introduction to McDonaldization.* Retrieved from http://www.Ritzer- cho1.qxd

RMHC. (2008). *Ronald McDonald House charities.* Retrieved from http:// www.rmhc.org//programs/rmhc-national-scholarship-program

RMHCSC. (2011). *Walk for kids 2011.* Retrieved from http://walk-forkids.org/faf/home/default.asp?ievent=446300

Robb, D. (2008, April). Nutritional information on restaurant menus – does it make any difference? *Health Habits.* Retrieved from http://www.healthhabits.ca/2009/04/01/nutritional-infor-mation-on-restaurant-menus-does-it-make-any-difference/-menus- does-it-make-any-difference/

Robert Wood Johnson Foundation. (2009). *Childhood obesity. Study suggests supermarket, fast- food restaurant location has little impact on children's weight.* Retrieved from http://www.rwjf.org/child-hoodobesity/digest.jsp?id=11166

Rodriguez, R. (2007, May 27). Employment: More seniors keep working after retirement. *Post-Gazette.com.* Retrieved from http://www.post-gazette.com/

Ronald McDonald House Charities. (2008a). *Ronald McDonald House.* Retrieved from http://rmhc.org/programs/ronald-mcdonald-house-program

Ronald McDonald House Charities. (2008b). *Ronald McDonald House Charities.* Retrieved from http://rmhc.org/about

Ronald McDonald House Charities. (2008c). *Helping families.* Retrieved from http://rmhc.org/families

Ronald McDonald House Charities. (2008d). *Ronald McDonald care mobile.* Retrieved from http://rmhc.org/programs/ronald-mcdonald-care-mobile-program

Ronald McDonald House Charities. (2008e). *Ronald McDonald family room.* Retrieved from http://rmhc.org/programs/ronald-mcdonald-family-room-program

Root, A.D., Toma, R.B., Frank, G.C., & Reiboldt, W. (2004). Meals identified as healthy choices on restaurant menus: an evaluation of accuracy [Abstract]. *Int J Food Sci Nutr.* 55(6): 449-54. Abstract retrieved from http://www.ncbi.nlm.nih.gov/pubmed/

Ruby Tuesday. (2012). *Nutritional menu guide.* Retrieved from http://www.rubytuesday.com/assets/menu/pdf/informational/nutrition.pdf

Rusk, K. (2008). San Jose committee to examine fast food ban. *Abc7news.* Retrieved from http://abclocal.go.com/kgo/story?section=news/local&id=6339125

Salary Stories. (2007, August 14) Fast food jobs: Salary of fast food workers. [Web log post]. Retrieved from http://blogs.payscale.com/salarystories/2007/08/fast-food-salar.html

Saletan, W. (2008, July). Food apartheid. Banning fast food in poor neighborhoods. *Slate Magazine.* Retrieved from http://www.slate.com/id/2196397/

Salkeld, L. (2012, May 24). How the 63 stone teenager who had to be cut from her home in £100,000 rescue gorged on junk food served up by her mum. *Online Mail.* Retrieved from http://www.dailymail.co.uk/news/article-2149609/Georgia-Davis-Britains-fattest-teenager-cut-home-hadnt-outdoors-6-months.html

Salkever, A. (2010, October). Why happy meals toys are controversial in California. *Daily Finance.* Retrieved from http://www.dailyfinance.com/2010/10/09/proposed-san-francisco-ban-on-happy-meals-toys-sparks-anger-from/

San Francisco happy meal toy ban takes effect, sidestepped by McDonald's. (2011, November 30). *Huffington Post.* Retrieved from http://www.huffingtonpost.com/2011/11/30 /san-francisco-happy-meal-ban_n_1121186.html

Santona, G. (Ed.). CSR world - McDonald's Corporation. *The European Lawyer.* Retrieved from http://www.europeanlawyer.co.uk/referencebooks_8_59.html

Scarborough Research. (2006). *Dining out is quintessentially American: The Scarborough Restaurant Report.* Retrieved from http://scarborough.com/press_releases/scarborough- restaurant-report-2006.pdf

Schlosser, E. (1998, September). Fast-food nation: The true cost of America's diet. *Rolling Stone Magazine, 794.* Retrieved from http://www.mcspotlight.org/media/press/ rollingstone1.html

Schlosser, E. (2002). *Fast food nation: The dark side of the all-American meal.* New York, NY: Perennial.

Schlosser, E. & Wilson, C. (2006). *Chew on this: Everything you don't know about fast food.* Boston, MA: Houghton Mifflin

Schoodoodle School Supplies Blog. (2011, April 7). *Are kids too plugged in? These statistics may get your attention.* Retrieved from http://www.schoodoodle.com/weblog/2011/04/07/ are-kids-too-plugged-in-these-statistics-may-get-your-attention/

Schreiner, B. (2008, October 1). Fast-food giant Yum Brands to start offering calorie information on menu boards in US. *Hartford Courant.* Retrieved from http://www.courant.com

ScienceDaily. (2007). *You're likely to order more calories at a 'healthy' restaurant.* Retrieved from http://www.sciencedaily.com/releases /2007/08/070829143638.htm

ScienceDaily. (2008). *Eating out can have both positive and negative impact on obesity.* Retrieved from http://www.sciencedaily.com/ releases/2008/01/080109094356.htm

Scott, M. (2010, September). New study: Obesity is bad for your bottom line. *Daily Finance.* Retrieved from http://64.12.68.155/story/ new-study-obesity-is-bad-for-your-bottom- line/19643116/

Sealey, G. (July 26). Obese man sues fast-food chains. *ABC News.* Retrieved from http://abcnews.go.com/US/story?id= 91427&page=1

Segway. (n.d.). *How the Segway PT works.* Retrieved from http:// www.segway.com/individual/learn-how-works.php

Sellers, P. (2011, August). McDonald's boss takes health crusade personally. *Fortune Magazine. Shine.*

Selvin, M. (2005, November 15). 'Cheeseburger bill' is high on menu in Washington. *Los Angeles Times.* Retrieved from http:// articles.com/2005/nov/15/business/fi-burger bill15

Sertl, B. (2011, April). Japanese Burger King launches meat monster: A 1,160 calorie burger. *Slashfood.* Retrieved from http://www.

slashfood.com/2011/04/13/japanese-burger-king- launches-meat-monster-a-1-160-calorie-burg/

Seventh-Day Adventist Dietetic Association. (n.d.). *"Good eating" guidelines*. Retrieved from http://www.sdada.org/eatingwell.htm

Severson, K. (2006, December 13). New York gets ready to count calories. *The New York Times*. Retrieved from http://www.nytimes.com

Severson, K. (2010, September 25). Told to eat its vegetables, America orders fries. *The New York Times*. Retrieved from http://www.nytimes.com/2010/09/25/health/policy/25vegetables.html?pagewanted=all

Sheeran, T.J. (2011, November). Ohio officials take 200-pound boy from mother. *Huffington Post.* Retrieved from http://www.huffingtonpost.com/2011/11/29/ohio-officials-take-200-p_n_1118186.html

Simmons, T. (2007, May 15). From fry cook to big cheese: McDonald's leader stars in ad. *The News & Observer.* Retrieved from http://www.newsobserver.com/print/tuesday/business/story/574244.html

Simon, P., Jarosz, C.J., Kuo, T., & Fielding, J.E. (2008, March). *Menu labeling as a potential strategy for combating the obesity epidemic. A health impact assessment.* Retrieved from http://www.euro.who.int/PAE/Gothenburgpaper.pdf

Simon, R. (2011, October 21). Easier nutrition ratings proposed for packages. *Los Angeles Times.*

Sinatra, S. (2006). *The fast food diet: Lose weight and feel great even if you're too busy to eat right.* Hoboken, NJ: John Wiley & Sons.

Smith, A. (2011, April). McDonald's to hire 50,000 workers – in 1 day. *CNN Money.* Retrieved from http://money.cnn.com/2011/04/04/news/companies/mcdonalds_jobs/index.htm

Smith, S.T. (2003, October 8). Fast-food chains attempt to help parents with healthy options. *Knight Ridder/Tribune Business News.* Retrieved from http://www.allbusiness.com

Spivack, M.S. (2007, May 16). Montgomery bans trans fats in restaurants, markets. *Washington Post.* Retrieved from http://www.washingtonpost.com

Spurlock, M. (Producer, Director). (2004). *Super size me.* [Documentary]. United States: Samuel Goldwyn Films.

Spurlock, M. (2006). *Don't eat this book: Fast food and the supersizing of America.* New York, NY: Berkley Books.

Spurlock, M. (2008, April 22). Eric Schlosser, Author of Fast Food Nation. *Guardian News & M36.asp*

Standora, L. (2005, January). Court leans on Mcd's in fat suit. *New York Daily News.* Retrieved from http://www.judicialaccountability.org/articles/mcdonaldcasedismissed .htm

Starbucks. (n.d.) *Nutrition by the Cup.*

Starbucks. (n.d.). *Nutrition by the Plate.*

Starbucks Coffee Company. (2008). *Company fact sheet.* Retrieved from http://www.news.starbucks.com/

Starnes, T. (2012, June). City wants to outlaw Coca Cola, sodas. *Fox News & Commentary.* Retrieved from http://radio.foxnews.com/toddstarnes/top-stories/city-wants-to-outlaw-coca- cola-sodas.html

State law banning trans fats from restaurants in effect. (2010, January). *KTVU News.* Retrieved from http://www.ktvu.com/news/22107348/detail.html

State University. (n.d.). *Ticket taker job description, career as a ticket taker, salary, employment -definition and nature of the work, education and training requirement, getting the job.* Retrieved October 2008 from http://careers.stateuniversity.com/pages/523/Ticket-Taker.html

Stein, J. (2009, August 19). What's on the menu? A dispute about menu labeling. *Los Angeles Times.* Retrieved from http://latimes-blogs.latimes.com/

Stein, J. (2011, June 22). We may be snacking more, but those extra calories might not be causing obesity. *Los Angeles Times.* Retrieved from http://www.latimes.com/

Stein, J. (2011, August 31). Half the people in U.S. drink sugary beverages daily, CDC says. *Los Angeles Times*. Retrieved from http://www.latimes.com/

Steinhauer, J. (2008, July 26). California bars restaurant use of trans fats. *The New York Times*. Retrieved from http://www.nytimes.com

Steinhauer, J. (2008, August 8). Fast-food curb meets with ambivalence in South Los Angeles. *The New York Times*. Retrieved from http://www.nytimes.com

Steintrager, M. (2010). Nutritionist-approved fast food. *Slashfood*. Retrieved from http://www.slashfood.com/2010/02/05/nutiritonist-approved-fast-food/

Sterrett, D. (2007, July). McDonald's faces teen labor shortage. *Workforce Management*. retrieved from http://www.workforce.com/section/00/article/25/01/75.html

Stokes, T. (2008, October 7). Many teens moving beyond burger flipping for employment. *Times Daily*. Retrieved from http://www.timesdaily.com

Story, M. & French, S. (2004). Food advertising and marketing directed at children and adolescents in the U.S. *International Journal of Behavioral Nutrition and Physical Activity*, 1(3).

Strom, S. (2011, November 30). Toys to cost extra in San Francisco happy meals. *The New York Times*. Retrieved from http://www.nytimes.com/

Strom, S. (2011, November 30). Toys stay in San Francisco happy meals, for a charge. *The New York Times*. Retrieved from http://www.nytimes.com/

Study questions accuracy of food labels. (2010, January). *ABC-WLS-TV*. Retrieved from http://abclocal.go.com/wls/story?section=news/health&id=7204556

SUBWAY. (2008a). *Restaurants History*. Retrieved from http://www.subway.com/subwayroot/AboutSubway/history/subwayHistory.aspx

SUBWAY. (2008b). *Helping society*. Retrieved from http://www.subway.com/subwayroot/ AboutSubway/helpingSociety/index.aspx

SUBWAY. (2008c). *Jared's statistics.* Retrieved from http://www.sub-way.com/subwayroot /MenuNutrition/Jared/jaredsStory.aspx

SUBWAY. (2011a). *Frequently asked questions.* Retrieved from http://www.subway.com/ StudentGuide/faq.htm

SUBWAY. (2011b). *SUBWAY FAQs.* Retrieved from http://www.subway.com/subwayroot /AboutSubway/subwayFaqs.aspx

Sutherland, A. (2009, August 17). NYC menu mayhem. *New York Post.* Retrieved from http://www.nypost.com/seven/08172009/news/regionalnews/nyc_menu_mahyem_184955

Sweet, L. (2010, May). Michelle Obama unveils anti-childhood obesity action plan. *Politics Daily.* Retrieved from http://www.politicsdaily.com/2010/05/11/michelle-obama-unveils-anti-childhood-obesity-action-plan/

Taco Bell. (2008). *Our company: history.* Retrieved from http://www.tacobell.com/

Taco Bell. (2012). *Nutrition info.* Retrieved from http://www.taco-bell.com/nutrition

Talwar, J. P. (2004). *Fast food, fast track: Immigrants, big business, and the American dream.* Boulder, CO: Westview Press.

Tanner, L. (2010, February). Girl's odyssey shows challenge of fighting obesity. *Yahoo! News.* Retrieved from http://news.yahoo.com/s/ap/20100201/ap_on_he_me/us_med_fighting_ obesity

Tanner, L. (2010, April). Bad habits can age you by 12 years, study suggests. *Yahoo! News.* Retrieved from http://news.yahoo.com/s/ap/us_med_bad_habits_survival

Taylor, A. (2011, May 8). Weight Watchers teams up with McDonald's, angering nutritionists. *Huffington Post.* Retrieved from http://www.huffingtonpost.com/2010/03/03/mcdonalds-teams-up-with-w_n_484061.html

Tecca. (2012, April). This Burger King whopper has so much bacon that it costs $80. *Yahoo News!* Retrieved from http://news.yahoo.com/blogs/technology-blog/burger-king-whopper-much-bacon-costs-80-220354571.html

Term-Papers.us (2005). *McDonald's.* Retrieved from http://www.term-papers.us/ts/bb/bmu 268.shtml

T.G.I. Fridays. (2012). *Nutritional information.* Retrieved from http://www.tgifridays.com/_images/pdfs/Nutritional.pdf

The Associated Press. (2010, October). Fast-food freebie ban gets ok in San Francisco. *Yahoo! News.* Retrieved from http://news.yahoo.com/s/ap/20101004/ap_on_bi_ge/us_fast_food_freebies

The Associated Press. (2012, June 12). Burger King rolls out summer BBQ sandwiches, bacon sundae. *USA Today.* Retrieved from http://www.usatoday.com/money/industries/food/story /2012-06-12/burger-king-limited-time-bbq-bacon-sundae/55552508/1

The most and least obese states in the U.S. (2012, March 2). *Huffington Post.* Retrieved from http://www.huffington-post.com/2012/03/02/obesity-in-united-states-statistics_n 1313297.html

Thompson, A. (2009, April 24). Family planning Ronald McDonald House benefit. *The Tifton Gazette.* Retrieved from http://www.tiftongazette.com

Today's Dietitian. (2011, July 27). McDonald's commitments to offer improved nutrition choices. [Electronic mailing list message]. Retrieved from todaysdietian@gvpub.com

Torrisi, L. (2012, April). Woman collapses at Heart Attack Grill. *ABC News.* Retrieved from http://abcnews.go.com/blogs/lifestyle/2012/04/woman-collapses-at-heart-attack-grill/

Trinidad, E. (2011, May 3). Taco Bell's cheesy double decker taco reviewed. *AOL News + Huffington Post.* Retrieved from http://www.huffingtonpost.com/

Tuberose. (n.d.). *Fast food.* [Web log post]. Retrieved from http://www.tuberose.com/Fast_Food.html

Tucker, T. (2011). McDonald's Corporation. *Answers.com.* Retrieved from http://www. answers.com/topic/mcdonald-s

Turner, B. (2009, May 3). Ronald McDonald House celebrates 20 years. *The Galveston County Daily News.* Retrieved from http://galvestondailynews.com

TV-Free America. *Television & health.* Retrieved from http://www.csun.edu/science/health/docs /tv&health.html

Tyler, R. (2009, August 13). Workers over 60 are surprise key to McDonald's sales. *Telegraph.co.uk.* Retrieved from http://www.telegraph.co.uk

U.S. Census Bureau. (2000a). *Percent of persons 25 years and over with bachelor's degree or higher.* Retrieved from http://factfinder.census.gov

U.S. Census Bureau. (2000b). *Educational attainment by sex: 2000.* Retrieved from www.census.gov/hhes/socdemo/education/data/cps/2000/tables.html

USDA. (2005). *Dietary guidelines for Americans 2005.* Retrieved from http://www.health.gov/dietaryguidelines/dga2005/recommendatins.htm

United States Department of Agrictulture. (2011a). *Dietary guidelines for Americans, 2010.* Retrieved from http://www.cnpp.usda.gov/dgas2010-policydocument.htm

United States Department of Agriculture. (2011b). *ChooseMyPlate.gov.* Retrieved from http://www.choosemyplate.gov/

U.S. Department of Health & Human Services. (2008a). *2008 Physical Activity Guidelines for Americans.* Retrieved from http://www.health.gov/paguidelines/

U.S. Department of Health & Human Services. (2008b). *Promoting healthy eating and physical activity for a healthier nation.* Retrieved from http://www.heathierus.gov

U.S. Department of Health & Human Services. (2012). *How to understand and use the nutrition facts label.* Retrieved from http://www.fda.gov/Food/ResourcesForYou/Consumers/NFLPM/ucm274593.htm

U.S. Department of Health & Human Services Wage and Hour Division. (2008). *Compliance assistance – fair labor standards act (FLSA).* Retrieved from http://www.dol.gov/esa/whd/flsa/

Vives, R. (2011, June 26). Swap soda for fresh fruit? No thanks, Angelenos say. *Los Angeles Times.* Retrieved from http://www.latimes.com/

References

Wald, J. (2003, February). McDonald's obesity suit tossed. *CNN Money*. Retrieved from http://money.cnn.com/2003/01/22/news/companies/mcdonalds/

Wald, J. (2003, February). Lawyers revise obesity lawsuit against McDonald's. *CNN*. Retrieved from http://www.cnn.com/2003/LAW/02/21/obesity.lawsuit/

Walke, H. (2010, October 20). Shocking ad links fast food and death. [Web log post]. *That's Fit*. Retrieved from http://www.thatsfit.com/2010/10/20/provocative-video-links-heart-disease-and-fast-food/

Walton, A. (2008, July 31). Committee approved ban on fast food in South L.A. *The Los Angeles Sentinel*. Retrieved from http://www.lasentinel.net

Warren, K. (2009). Reading the fine print: A variety of technologies helps restaurant comply with menu-labeling laws. *QSR Magazine*. Retrieved from http://qsrmagazine.com/articles/tools/121/menu-labeling-1.phtml

Warshaw, H.S. (2005). *Guide to healthy restaurant eating* (3rd ed.). Alexandria, VA: American Diabetes Association.

Warshaw, H.S. (2008). *Eat out, eat right* (3rd ed.). Chicago, IL: Surrey Books.

Warshaw, H.S. (2006). *Guide to healthy fast-food eating*. Alexandria, VA: American Diabetes Association

Wass, N. (2102, January 11). Hungry for another title, Revens' Lewis watches diet. *USA Today*. Retrieved from http://www.usatoday.com/

Watson, G. (2012, February). Cassanove McKinzy spurned Clemson because he missed the Chick-fil-A. [Web log post]. Retrieved from http://sports.yahoo.com/blogs/ncaaf-dr-saturday/cassanova-mckinzy-spurned-clemson-because-didn-t-chick-015506961.html

Watson, S. (2008, May). State says hundred of 9/11 rescue workers now dead, admits undercount. *Infowars.net*. Retrieved from http://www.infowars.net/articles/may2008/090508 Workers.htm

Weight Watchers teams up with McDonald's, angering nutrition-ists [Web log post]. (2010, March 3). *Huffington Post*. Retrieved from http://www.huffingtonpost.com/2010/03/03/mcdonalds-teams-up-with-w_n_484061.html

Weintraub, L. (2011, April). McDonald's holds "national hiring day" for 50,000 potential employees. *The Vista*. Retrieved from http://www.theusdvista.com

Weise, E. (2011, December 6). Beware the sugar in cereals marketed to kids. *USA Today*. Retrieved from http://www.usatoday.com/

Weiser, B. (2003, January). Big Macs can make you fat? No kidding, a judge rules. *New York Times*. Retrieved from http://www.judicialaccountability.org/articles/mcdonaldscasedismissed.htm

Wendy's. (2008a). *Dave Thomas*. Retrieved from http://www.wendys.com/dave/davethomas_biography.pdf

Wendy's. (2008b). *The Wendy's story*. Retrieved from http://www.wendy's.com/about_us/story.jsp

Wendy's. (2008c). *Corporate responsibility*. Retrieved from http://www.aboutwendy's.com/ /Responsibility/

Wendy's. (2008d). *Wendy's kicks off 15th high school Heisman*. Retrieved from http://www.wendys.com/about_us/news/index.jsp

Wendy's. (2012). *Nutrition information*. Retrieved from http://www.wendys.com/food /pdf/us/nutrition.pdf

Wexler, S. (2008, August). Fat Chance: A ban on new fast-food restaurants in south Los_Angeles doesn't address the real causes of obesity. *The American*. Retrieved from http://www.american.com/archive/2008/august-08-08/fast-chance/

Whaley, S. (2004, July). Downsized at McDonald's; filmmaker loses 18 pounds in debunking fast-food flick. *Competitive Enterprise Institute*. Retrieved from http://cei.org/op-eds-and-articles/downsized-mcdonalds-filmmaker-loses-18-pounds-debunking-fast-food-flick

What Consumers Think. (2008, June). In the last 60 days, how often have you eaten at fine dining restaurants? *QSR Magazine.com*. Retrieved from http://www.qsrmagazine.com/articles/features/116/consumer_charts/8.3

What Consumers Think. (2008, June). Do you agree that, on the whole, fast-food menus have gotten healthier over the past 3 years? *QSR Magazine*. Retrieved from http://www.qsrmagazine.com/articles/features/116/consumer_charts/26.1

What Consumers Think. (2008, June). In the last 60 days, how often have you eaten at fast food restaurants? *QSR Magazine*. Retrieved from http://www.qsrmagazine.com/articles/features/116/consumer_charts/8.1

White, E. (2009, August). Q and A with author Julie Powell. *Oprah.com*. Retrieved from http://www.oprah.com/food/Q-and-A-with-Julie-and-Julia-Author-Julie-Powell

White, M.C. (2009, August 3). McMoonshine? Fast-food outlets add booze to menus. *Daily Finance*. Retrieved from http://www.dailyfinance.com/2009/08/03/mcmoonshine-fast-food-outlets-add-booze-to-menus/

Whitman, W. (2009, May). Former crew employee oversees more than 5,000 restaurants in 21 states. *Business Opportunities Journal*. Retrieved from http://www.boj.com/articles/franchise/mcdonalds_king.htm

Williams, W. (2005, November). McJobs: dead end jobs? *Capitalism Magazine*. Retrieved from http://www.capmag.com/articles.asp?ID=4487

Williamson, D. (2003, January). UNC study confirms that food portion sizes increased in U.S. over two decades. *UNC News Services*. Retrieved from http://www.unc.edu/news/archives/jan03/popkin011603.html

Wilson, C. (2011, August 23). Final word: Getting in deep (fried) at the state fair. Retrieved from http://www.usatoday.com/

Wilson, T.V. (n.d). How fast food works. *TLC Cooking "The History of Fast Food."* Retrieved from http://recipes.howstuffworks.com/fast-food3.htm

Winfield, N. (2010, February). Italy minister defends boost for McDonald's burger. *Yahoo! News*. Retrieved from http://news.yahoo.com/s/ap_travel/eu_travel_brief_ital_mcitaly

Winterman, D. (2008, February). The towns where people live the longest. *BBC News.* Retrieved from http://news.bbc.co.uk/2/hi/uk_news/magazine/7250675.stm

Wood, L. (1987, July). Poll: Teens still enjoy fast-food work. *Nation's Restaurant News.* Retrieved from http://findarticles.com/p/articles/mi_m3190/is_/ai_5102385

Wong, W.Y. (2009, April). Eat out healthy: How to manage weight when eating outside the home. *Suite101.com.* Retrieved from http://weightloss.suite101.com/article.cfm/eat_out_healthily

World Health Organization. (n.d.). *Food security.* Retrieved from http://www.who.int/trade/glossary/story028/en/

Wouters, J. (2010, September). McDonald's happy meal charity promo goes easy on the cash. *Walletpop.* Retrieved from http://www.walletpop.com

Wright, W., & Middendorf, G. (Eds.). (2008). *The fight over food: Producers, consumers, and activists challenge the global food system.* University Park, PA: The Pennsylvania State University Press.

Yamamoto, J.A., Yamamoto, J.B., Yamamoto, B.E., & Yamamoto, L.G. (2004). Adolescent fast food and restaurant ordering behavior with and without calorie and fat content menu information. *Journal of Adolescent Health, 37,* 397-402. doi: 10.1016/j.jadohealth.2004.10_.002.

Yamamoto, J.A., Yamamoto, J.B., Yamamoto, B.E., & Yamamoto L.G. (2006). Adolescent calorie/fat menu ordering at fast food restaurants compared to other restaurants. *Hawaii Med J,* 65(8), 231-6.

Yamamoto, J. (2007, September 26). Only 29 percent of Americans have a college degree. *The Olympian.* Retrieved from http://www.theolympian.com/209/story/227366.html

York, E.B. (2012, March 22). McDonald's chief Jim Skinner to retire: Don Thompson, president and chief operating officer, named successor. *Chicago Tribune.* Retrieved from http://articles.chicagotribune.com/2012-03-22/site/ct-biz-0322-mcdonalds-skinner-   20120322_1_ceo-jim-cantalupo-mcdonald-s-usa-mcdonald-s-plan

Yum! Brands Foundation. (2008a). *About Yum! Brands.* Retrieved from http://www.yum.com/ about/default.asp

Yum! Brands Foundation. (2008b). *Yum! Brands Foundation.* Retrieved from http://www.yum.com/responsibility/foundation.asp

Yum! Brands, Inc. (2008c). *International philanthropy.* Retrieved from http://www.yum.com/responsibility/intphil.asp

Yum! Brands, Inc. (2008d). *Global diversity community.* Retrieved from http://www.yum.com/responsibility/div_community.asp

Yum! Brands, Inc. (2008e). *The Pizza Hut Book It! program.* Retrieved from http://www.yum.com/responsibility/bookit.asp

Yum! Brands, Inc. (2008f). *The KFC colonel's scholars.* Retrieved from http://www.yum.com/responsibility/colscholars.asp

Yum! Brands, Inc. (2008g). *The Taco Bell teen programs.* Retrieved from http://www.yum.com/responsibility/teenprograms.asp

Yum! Brands, Inc. (2008h). *World hunger relief week global initiative.* Retrieved from http://www.yum.com/responsibility/hungerrelief.asp

Yum! Brands, Inc. (2008i). *The YUMeals program.* Retrieved from http://www.yum.com/responsibility/yumeals.asp

Zientek, H. (2009, March 27). McDonald's offer 'work trials' to unemployed. *Huddersfield Daily Examiner.* Retrieved from http://findarticles.com/p/articles/mi_6784/is_2009_March_27/ai_n31482987?

Zinczenko, D., Goulding, M. & Murrow, L. (with). (n.d.). 16 secrets the restaurant industry doesn't want you to know. *Men's Health.* Retrieved from http://www.menshealth.com/16secrets/secretchains.html

Zinczenko, D., & Goulding, M. (with). (2008). *Eat this not that!* New York, NY: Rodale, Inc.

Zinczenko, D., & Goulding, M.(with). (2008). *Eat this not that! For kids!* New York, NY: Rodale, Inc.

Zinczenko, D. & Goulding M. (with). (2009). *Eat this not that!* New York, NY: Rodale, Inc.

Zinczenko, D., & Goulding, M. (with). (2010). *Drink this not that!* New York, NY: Rodale, Inc.

Zinczenko, D., & Goulding, M. (with). (2010). *Cook this not that!* New York, NY: Rodale, Inc.

Zinczenko D., & Goulding, M. (with). (2010). *Eat this not that, Restaurant survival guide.* New York, NY: Rodale, Inc.

Zinczenko, D. & Goulding, M. (with). (2011) *Eat this not that!* New York, NY: Rodale, Inc.

Zuber, A. (2001, May). A career in foodservice: High turnover. *Nation's Restaurant News.* Retrieved from http://findarticles.com/p/articles/mi_m3190/is_21_35/ai_75100597

Zwillich, T. (2005, October). House votes to ban 'obesity' lawsuits' against fast food industry. *FoxNews.com.* Retrieved from http://www.foxnews.com/story/0,2933,172805,00.html

17974372R00141

Made in the USA
Lexington, KY
12 October 2012